Effective GP Commissioning – Essential Knowledge, Skills and Attitudes

A practical guide

SUNIL GUPTA

General Practitioner
Chair, Professional Executive Committee
NHS South East Essex
Joint Clinical Director, Castle Point GP Consortium, Essex

Foreword by

SIMON GREGORY

Postgraduate Dean, East of England
General Practitioner, Northampton

Radcliffe Publishing
London • New York

Radcliffe Publishing Ltd
33–41 Dallington Street
London
EC1V 0BB
United Kingdom

www.radcliffepublishing.com
Electronic catalogue and worldwide online ordering facility.

British Library Cataloguing in Publication Data

A catalogue record for this book is available from the British Library.

ISBN-13: 978 184619 520 4

The paper used for the text pages of this book is FSC® certified. FSC® (The Forest Stewardship Council®) is an international network to promote responsible management of the world's forests.

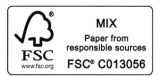

MIX
Paper from
responsible sources
FSC
www.fsc.org
FSC® C013056

Typeset by Pindar NZ, Auckland, New Zealand
Printed and bound by TJI Digital, Padstow, Cornwall, UK

Contents

Foreword

The National Health Service (NHS) White Paper *Equity and Excellence: liberating the NHS* has proposed that general practitioners (GPs) working together in clusters or consortia will commission the bulk of NHS care for the populations they serve. The spectrum of reaction to this has varied from abhorrence that GPs may be involved in rationing decisions to early adopters rushing to begin the task. In reality GPs have been involved in such decisions for many years. It is vital to the doctor–patient relationship that the individual patient in the consultation can rely upon their physician making their care the utmost priority, but doctors have always balanced this with population responsibility and appropriate use of resources. We have always, I suggest, applied this to our prescribing and referrals, and to the resources of our own practices. GPs have a history of successful involvement in and taking responsibility for commissioning decisions through locality commissioning groups, fundholding, practice-based commissioning (PBC) group and primary care trust (PCT) professional executive committees and boards and practice-based commissioning. But these reforms bring much greater responsibility and the requirement that all GPs participate. Whilst the 'consortia' are likely to be run by enthusiasts, all GPs will need an understanding of what is being done in their name and will share accountability.

This book provides a useful resource for all GPs whatever their level of engagement and, indeed, also for non-clinicians. Sunil Gupta is clearly a business magpie as well as a GP, and he has an incredible ability to gather, organise and present useful information. This book is well-researched, linking considerable volumes of information in a useful, constructive manner. He moves from considering what commissioning is and the role of leadership, to considering the knowledge, skills and attitudes required. Along the way he takes much of our current knowledge, such as our consultation skills, and place this in the commissioning context. To his great credit, Sunil Gupta is also prepared to make some unpalatable suggestions that, whilst may seem unacceptable or unachievable, do stimulate thought, may trigger debate and generate new mindsets.

Healthcare inflation far outstrips the economy and public expectations continue to rise. We can be in no doubt that the challenge ahead is vast and that each of us is going to be involved in making some very tough decisions, which we will have to justify to the populations we serve – indeed, to individual patients and their loved ones. The difficult task is maintaining our integrity and the integrity of the doctor–patient relationship whilst commissioning with an ever-more-restricted budget and ever-increasing demand. To achieve this we will need the assistance of our patients and the wider NHS workforce. Working with these other parties is something that GPs already do and can continue to do. The challenge is vast and the risks high. We need support and resources to do this. Sunil Gupta's book is one such resource.

Professor Simon Gregory
Postgraduate Dean, East of England
General Practitioner, Northampton
January 2011

Preface

The NHS White Paper of July 2010, *Equity and Excellence: liberating the NHS*, has proposed a massive shake up of the National Health Service (NHS) in England.[1] The primary care trusts will be abolished and their commissioning function, it is proposed, is to be mainly taken over by general practitioners (GPs) working together in consortia. This has been viewed with excitement by some GPs, but others worry that they do not have the knowledge and skills to take on the task of commissioning on such a large scale.

This book is intended to help clinicians and non-clinicians involved in GP commissioning succeed in this difficult task. It is in four main parts. Part 1 covers commissioning. Parts 2, 3 and 4 discuss some of the knowledge, skills and attitudes required for effective GP commissioning.

Part 1 outlines what commissioning is and how it is done. It also outlines the *Medical Leadership Competency Framework*, which describes the competencies doctors need to be more actively involved in the planning, delivery and transformation of services. There is also a discussion of the financial and political environment facing the NHS, as well as the government's plans. It ends with ideas – some of which will be controversial – about how to save money in the NHS.

Part 2 discusses some of the knowledge needed for effective GP commissioning. It ranges from topics that will be familiar to doctors, like long-term conditions management, patient safety and the wider determinants of health, to many topics never taught at medical schools or in postgraduate education. These include delegation, productivity and the financial accounts. Also outlined are some management theories as well the meaning of common terms used in commissioning.

Part 3 discusses some of the skills needed for effective GP commissioning. These range from assertiveness to innovation, from negotiating to presentational and from media skills to emotional competence. Again many of these topics are never taught to clinicians, but they make a significant difference to a person's effectiveness in a commissioning role.

Part 4 of this book describes some of the attitudes needed for effective GP commissioning. It begins with the Nolan Principles of public life (selflessness, integrity, objectivity, accountability, openness, honesty and leadership).

I have tried to bring together in this book a large number of helpful ideas and concepts from literally hundreds of people from many diverse fields such as management, leadership, psychology, medicine, philosophy, education, self-development, accountancy and economics. I have done my best to name the originators of these ideas but I would like to apologise in advance to any person who has not been given appropriate credit for their original thoughts. These ideas and concepts are needed because the NHS is going to face very difficult challenges in the years ahead. I hope this book will contribute to the NHS successfully meeting these challenges.

Sunil Gupta
January 2011

REFERENCE

1 NHS and Department of Health. *Equity and Excellence: liberating the NHS*. White Paper, Cm 7881. Norwich: The Stationery Office; 2010.

About the author

Dr Sunil Gupta has been a GP in Essex since 1995. For the last three years he has been Chair of the Professional Executive Committee of NHS South East Essex. He has recently taken on the role of Joint Clinical Director of a PBC group. His other roles include GP trainer, course organiser, examiner for the Royal College of General Practitioners and a member of the Fitness to Practise Panel of the General Medical Council. He is particularly interested in improving patient safety and is a member of the East of England Clinical Programme Board for Patient Safety.

To Molly, Shubham and Naman

PART 1

Commissioning

CHAPTER 1

What is commissioning?

Commissioning is the process of assessing the needs of a local population and putting in place services to meet those needs.

PROCESS OF HEALTHCARE COMMISSIONING

1 Assess the healthcare needs of the local population and review how well existing service provision meets those needs.
2 Identify priorities for investment and design services/identify opportunities to meet the needs.
3 Acquire these services/create opportunities through contracts with a variety of service providers including GPs, NHS trusts, foundation trusts, third sector and independent sector organisations and partnerships with other agencies.
4 Ensure the services are provided effectively, and monitor quality and outcomes.

WHY DO WE NEED COMMISSIONERS?

➤ To act as advocates for patients and improve patient care, patient experience and service responsiveness and performance.
➤ To act as custodians for taxpayers by improving efficiency and value for money.
➤ To ensure NHS planning and provision is needs/demand-led, not supplier-led and to bring about reconfiguration of services by shifting investment.
➤ To improve patient safety.
➤ To improve health outcomes.

THE WORLD CLASS COMMISSIONING PROGRAMME

Launched in December 2007, this programme aimed to drive up the commissioning capability of local NHS commissioners. It introduced 11 organisational competencies that set out the knowledge, skills, behaviours and characteristics commissioners need:

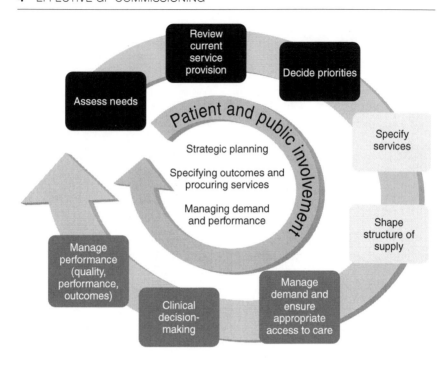

FIGURE 1.1 The commissioning cycle.

1   locally lead the NHS
2   work with community partners
3   engage with public and patients
4   collaborate with clinicians
5   manage knowledge and assess needs
6   prioritise investment
7   stimulate the market
8   promote improvement and innovation
9   secure procurement skills
10 manage the local health system
11 make sound financial investments.

THE APPROACH OF THIS BOOK

I believe that the knowledge, skills and attitudes needed for effective GP commissioning are similar to the competences of World Class Commissioning but not identical. These requirements are covered in Parts 2–4:

Part 2 Knowledge needed for effective GP commissioning

➤ Assessing local health needs.
➤ Budgets.

➤ Business plans.
➤ Change implementation.
➤ Commissioning case checklist.
➤ Decision-making.
➤ Delegation.
➤ Effective use of emails.
➤ Ethics.
➤ Financial accounts.
➤ Integration.
➤ Key Terms.
➤ Long-term conditions management.
➤ Management theories.
➤ Mentoring.
➤ Patient safety.
➤ Public involvement and patient engagement.
➤ Procurement.
➤ Productivity.
➤ Project management.
➤ Quality improvement.
➤ Recruitment.
➤ Teamwork.
➤ Wider determinants of health.

Part 3 Skills needed for effective GP commissioning

➤ Assertiveness.
➤ Avoiding burnout.
➤ Cognitive behavioural therapy skills.
➤ Conflict resolution.
➤ Communication skills.
➤ Consultation skills.
➤ Dealing with difficult colleagues.
➤ Emotional Bank Account.
➤ Emotional competence.
➤ Innovation.
➤ Media skills.
➤ Meetings skills.
➤ Negotiating skills.
➤ People skills.
➤ Planning skills.
➤ Political skills.
➤ Presentational skills.
➤ Stress management.
➤ Time management.

Part 4 Attitudes needed for effective GP commissioning

➤ Adherence to the Nolan Principles of public life (selflessness, integrity, objectivity, accountability, openness, honesty and leadership).

➤ Other attitudes needed for effective GP commissioning (cost-effectiveness, long-term thinking, outcomes not activity, patient focus, pragmatism not ideology, tough love and a commitment to creating win-win situations).

SUMMARY

➤ Healthcare commissioning is the process of assessing the needs of a local population and putting in place services to meet those needs.

➤ A large range of knowledge, skills and attitudes are required to carry out effective healthcare commissioning.

CHAPTER 2

The *Medical Leadership Competency Framework*

This framework describes the leadership competences that doctors need in order to become more actively involved in the planning, delivery and transformation of health services.

It has been jointly developed by the Academy of Medical Royal Colleges and the NHS Institute for Innovation and Improvement in conjunction with others.

The framework can be used to highlight individual strengths and development areas through self-assessment and structured feedback from colleagues as well as assist with personal development planning and career progression.

The framework is in five parts:

1 Personal Qualities
2 Working with Others
3 Managing Services
4 Improving Services
5 Setting Direction.

PERSONAL QUALITIES

Doctors showing effective leadership need to draw upon their values, strengths and abilities to deliver high standards of care.

This requires doctors to demonstrate competence in:

➤ Self-awareness: being aware of their own values, principles, assumptions, and by being able to learn from experiences.
➤ Self-management: organising and managing themselves while taking account of the needs and priorities of others.
➤ Self-development: learning through participating in continuing professional development and from experience and feedback.
➤ Acting with integrity: behaving in an open and ethical manner.

WORKING WITH OTHERS

Doctors show effective leadership by working with others in teams and networks to deliver and improve services.

This requires doctors to demonstrate competence in:

➤ Developing networks: working in partnership with colleagues within and across systems and improving services.
➤ Building and maintaining relationships: listening, supporting others, gaining trust and showing understanding.
➤ Encouraging contribution: creating an environment where others have the opportunity to contribute.
➤ Working within teams: to deliver and improve services.

MANAGING SERVICES

Doctors showing effective leadership are focused on the success of the organisation(s) in which they work.

This requires doctors to demonstrate competence in:

➤ Planning: actively contributing to plans to achieve service goals.
➤ Managing resources: knowing what resources are available and using their influence to ensure that resources are used efficiently and safely.
➤ Managing people: providing direction, reviewing performance and motivating others.
➤ Managing performance: holding themselves and others accountable for service outcomes.

IMPROVING SERVICES

Doctors showing effective leadership make a real difference to people's health by delivering high-quality services and by developing improvements to services.

This requires doctors to demonstrate competence in:

➤ Ensuring patient safety: assessing and managing risk to patients associated with service improvement.
➤ Critically evaluating: being able to think analytically, conceptually and to identify where services can be improved.
➤ Encouraging innovation: creating a climate of continuous service improvement.
➤ Facilitating transformation: actively contributing to change processes that lead to improving healthcare.

SETTING DIRECTION

Doctors showing effective leadership contribute to the vision and aspirations of their organisation and act in a manner consistent with its values.

This requires doctors to demonstrate competence in:

➤ Identifying the contexts for change: being aware of the range of factors to be taken into account.

➤ Applying knowledge and evidence: gathering information to produce an evidence-based challenge to systems and processes in order to identify opportunities for service improvements.

➤ Making decisions: integrating values with evidence to inform decisions.

➤ Evaluating Impact: measuring and evaluating outcomes, taking corrective action where necessary and by being held to account for their decisions.

SUMMARY

➤ The *Medical Leadership Competency Framework* describes the leadership competencies that doctors need to become more actively involved in the planning, delivery and transformation of health services.

➤ It is made up of five areas: Personal Qualities, Working with Others, Managing Services, Improving Services and Setting Direction.

REFERENCE

Academy of Medical Royal Colleges and NHS Institute for Innovation and Improvement. *Medical Leadership Competency Framework*: enhancing engagement in medical leadership. 3rd ed. Coventry: NHS Institute for Innovation and Improvement; 2010.

CHAPTER 3

The financial environment

The NHS budget has increased over the last decade by over 6% a year, in real terms. This increased funding has enabled the NHS to expand the workforce, raise salaries, improve and update its equipment and infrastructure and deliver more care to more people more quickly.

In the financial year 2009/10, the UK recorded general government net borrowing of £159.8 billion, which was equivalent to 11.4% of the gross domestic product (GDP). At the end of March 2010 general government debt was £1000.4 billion, equivalent to 71.3% of GDP.

As a result of the financial situation of the country, the NHS will face very difficult financial circumstances in the next few years. The Comprehensive Spending Review for the NHS in England announced in October 2010 that funding will rise by £10 billion to £114 billion over the next four years – the equivalent of a 0.1% a year increase in real terms. This increase will be easily swallowed by rising costs from factors such as obesity and the ageing population.

The NHS will have to make between £15 billion and £20 billion of efficiency savings by 2015, which is equivalent to about 4% productivity gains each year.

SUMMARY

➤ Because of the financial situation of the country, the NHS will face very difficult financial circumstances in the next few years.

CHAPTER 4

The political environment

Over the last few years, NHS policies have contributed to three main government policy aims.
1   Improve patient care and in particular reduce inequalities in access to care.
2   Improve the patient's experience of services.
3   Achieve better value for money.

To try to achieve these policy aims, four types of reforms have been carried out.
1   Demand-side reforms: more choice and a much stronger voice for patients.

2   Supply-side reforms: more diverse providers, with more freedom to innovate and improve services.

3   Transactional reforms: money following the patients, rewarding the best and most efficient providers, giving others the incentive to improve.

4   System Management reforms: a framework of system management, regulation and decision making which guarantees safety and quality, fairness, equity and value for money.

SUMMARY
➤ Over the past few years NHS policy has been directed at improving patient care, improving the patient's experience of services and achieving better value for money.

REFERENCE
British Thoracic Society. *Jargon Buster*. British Thoracic Society Reports. 2010; 2(1).

CHAPTER 5

Government plans

EQUITY AND EXCELLENCE: LIBERATING THE NHS, JULY 2010[1]

Our strategy for the NHS: an executive summary

1 The Government upholds the values and principles of the NHS: of a comprehensive service, available to all, free at the point of use and based on clinical need, not the ability to pay.

2 We will increase health spending in real terms in each year of this Parliament.

3 Our goal is an NHS which achieves results that are amongst the best in the world.

Putting patients and public first

4 We will put patients at the heart of the NHS, through an information revolution and greater choice and control.

   a Shared decision-making will become the norm: no decision about me without me.

   b Patients will have access to the information they want, to make choices about their care. They will have increased control over their own care records.

   c Patients will have choice of any provider, choice of consultant-led team, choice of GP practice and choice of treatment. We will extend choice in maternity through new maternity networks.

   d The Government will enable patients to rate hospitals and clinical departments according to the quality of care they receive, and we will require hospitals to be open about mistakes and always tell patients if something has gone wrong.

   e The system will focus on personalised care that reflects individuals' health and care needs, supports carers and encourages strong joint arrangements and local partnerships.

   f We will strengthen the collective voice of patients and the public through arrangements led by local authorities, and at national level, through a powerful Commission.

g   We will seek to ensure that everyone, whatever their need or background, benefits from these arrangements.

Improving healthcare outcomes

5   To achieve our ambition for world-class healthcare outcomes, the service must be focused on outcomes and the quality standards that deliver them. The Government's objectives are to reduce mortality and morbidity, increase safety, and improve patient experience and outcomes for all:

a   The NHS will be held to account against clinically credible and evidence-based outcome measures, not process targets. We will remove targets with no clinical justification.

b   A culture of open information, active responsibility and challenge will ensure that patient safety is put above all else, and that failings such as those in Mid-Staffordshire cannot go undetected.

c   Quality standards, developed by NICE, will inform the commissioning of all NHS care and payment systems. Inspection will be against essential quality standards.

d   We will pay drug companies according to the value of new medicines, to promote innovation, ensure better access for patients to effective drugs and improve value for money. As an interim measure, we are creating a new Cancer Drug Fund, which will operate from April 2011; this fund will support patients to get the drugs their doctors recommend.

e   Money will follow the patient through transparent, comprehensive and stable payment systems across the NHS to promote high-quality care, drive efficiency, and support patient choice.

f   Providers will be paid according to their performance. Payment should reflect outcomes, not just activity, and provide an incentive for better quality.

Autonomy, accountability and democratic legitimacy

6   The Government's reforms will empower professionals and providers, giving them more autonomy and, in return, making them more accountable for the results they achieve, accountable to patients through choice and accountable to the public at local level:

a   The forthcoming Health Bill will give the NHS greater freedoms and help prevent political micromanagement.

b   The Government will devolve power and responsibility for commissioning services to the healthcare professionals closest to patients: GPs and their practice teams working in consortia.

c   To strengthen democratic legitimacy at local level, local authorities will promote the joining up of local NHS services, social care and health improvement.

d   We will establish an independent and accountable NHS Commissioning

Board. The Board will lead on the achievement of health outcomes, allocate and account for NHS resources, lead on quality improvement and promoting patient involvement and choice. The Board will have an explicit duty to promote equality and tackle inequalities in access to healthcare. We will limit the powers of Ministers over day-to-day NHS decisions.

e   We aim to create the largest social enterprise sector in the world by increasing the freedoms of foundation trusts and giving NHS staff the opportunity to have a greater say in the future of their organisations, including as employee-led social enterprises. All NHS trusts will become or be part of a foundation trust.

f   Monitor will become an economic regulator, to promote effective and efficient providers of health and care, to promote competition, regulate prices and safeguard the continuity of services.

g   We will strengthen the role of the Care Quality Commission as an effective quality inspectorate across both health and social care.

h   We will ring-fence the public health budget, allocated to reflect relative population health outcomes, with a new health premium to promote action to reduce health inequalities.

Cutting bureaucracy and improving efficiency

7   The NHS will need to achieve unprecedented efficiency gains, with savings reinvested in front-line services, to meet the current financial challenge and the future costs of demographic and technological change:

a   The NHS will release up to £20 billion of efficiency savings by 2014, which will be reinvested to support improvements in quality and outcomes.

b   The Government will reduce NHS management costs by more than 45% over the next four years, freeing up further resources for front-line care.

c   We will radically delayer and simplify the number of NHS bodies, and radically reduce the Department of Health's own NHS functions. We will abolish quangos that do not need to exist and streamline the functions of those that do.

Conclusion: making it happen

8   We will maintain constancy of purpose. This White Paper[1] is the long-term plan for the NHS in this Parliamentary term and beyond. We will give the NHS a coherent, stable, enduring framework for quality and service improvement. The debate on health should no longer be about structures and processes, but about priorities and progress in health improvement for all.

9   This is a challenging and far-reaching set of reforms, which will drive cultural changes in the NHS. We are setting out plans for managing change, including the transitional roles of strategic health authorities and primary care trusts. Implementation will happen bottom-up.

Many of the commitments made in the White Paper of which this is an executive summary require primary legislation and are subject to Parliamentary approval.[1]

SUMMARY

➤ The NHS White Paper of July 2010[1] proposes changes that the government hopes will put patients and public first, improve healthcare outcomes, improve autonomy, accountability and democratic legitimacy.
➤ It also hopes to cut bureaucracy and improve efficiency in the NHS.

REFERENCE

1 NHS and Department of Health. *Equity and Excellence: liberating the NHS*. White Paper, Cm 7881. Norwich: The Stationery Office; 2010. pp. 3–6.

CHAPTER 6

Quality, innovation, productivity and prevention

In response to financial challenges, the Department of Health has established quality, innovation, productivity and prevention (QIPP) as the guiding principles to help the NHS deliver its quality and efficiency commitments. QIPP is working at a national, regional and local level to support clinical teams and NHS organisations to improve the quality of care they deliver while making efficiency savings that can be reinvested in the service to deliver year-on-year quality improvements.

QIPP is trying to engage NHS staff to lead and support change. At a regional and local level there are QIPP plans which address the quality and productivity challenge, and these are supported by the national QIPP workstreams which are producing tools and programmes to help local change leaders in successful implementation.

There are 12 national workstreams in total. Five deal broadly with how the NHS commission care, covering long-term conditions, right care, safe care, urgent care and end of life care. Five deal with how the NHS run, staff and supply its organisations, covering productive care (staff productivity), non-clinical procurement, medicines use and procurement, efficient back office functions and pathology rationalisation. There are two enabling workstreams covering primary care commissioning and contracting and the role of digital technology in delivering quality and productivity improvement.

THE 12 WORKSTREAMS
Commissioning and pathways
1 Safe care

Aims:
➤ 80% reduction in hospital acquired pressure ulcers (grade 3–4)
➤ 30% reduction in community acquired pressure ulcers (grade 3–4)
➤ 50% reduction in catheter-acquired urinary tract infections
➤ 25% reduction in falls in care.[1]

2 Right care

Aim: [T]o change thinking on commissioning care away from organisations and contracts to commissioning high value, whole system pathways, underpinned by networks rather than institutions and putting the citizen and the patient at the centre of this discussion . . . A key component is the provision of tools and analysis which highlight the often large and unexplained variations in spend on healthcare and health outcomes for the commissioner's population.[1]

3 Long-term conditions

Aim: [T]o deliver a national support and improvement programme that will support local geographic areas to implement a generic model for supporting patients with LTCs [long-term conditions] based on four key principles.

1 Commissioners understanding the needs of their population and managing those at risk to prevent disease progression.
2 Empowering patients to maximise self-management including ensuring patients have a care plan and appropriate information and knowledge about how to manage their condition.
3 Providing joined-up and personal services particularly in community and primary care and working closely and effectively with social care.
4 Strong professional and clinical leadership and workforce development.[1]

4 Urgent care

Aims: [T]o maximise the number of instances when the right care is given by the right person at the right place and right time for patients. The workstream starts from a perspective that rather than 'educating' patients about where it is appropriate for them to go, we should focus on designing a simple system that guides them to where they should go.

It aims to achieve a 10% reduction in the number of patients attending Accident and Emergency with associated reductions in ambulance journeys and admissions.[1]

5 End of life care

Aim: The workstream will focus on better identifying and putting care plans in place for high-risk groups of patients – such as those in residential and nursing homes. The workstream will offer the NHS:

➤ changing national levers to support good end of life care
➤ developing and testing questions that clinicians can ask to best identify patients nearing the end of life
➤ support to NHS organisations so that they can review their cohort of end of life care patients and management of this – e.g. clinical dashboards; reviewing unplanned/unexpected deaths
➤ support to SHAs [strategic health authorities] to challenge PCT investment plans for community end of life care services
➤ identifying organisations that can be sites for rapid improvement and

facilitate sharing of learning via website and events
➤ disseminating best practice and tools that have been developed as part of the End of Life care strategy – e.g. elearning module on communications.[1]

Provider efficiency

6 Back office efficiency and optimal management

Aims:
➤ High-level guidance to pilot sites on key issues for change and ways to resolution.
➤ High-level programme/project monitoring to pilot sites and guidance with specific issues.
➤ Sign-posting of resources where additional support may be obtained to local implementations.
➤ Additional change support from central bodies such as NHS institute, commercial directorate, etc. if required.
➤ Clear communication of opportunities and products that can reinforce their regional plans through SHAs.[1]

7 Procurement

Aims:
➤ A best practice procurement checklist to ensure maximum local efficiency.
➤ Development and implementation of procurement tools to increase transparency and drive cost improvement (reverse auctions, etc.).[1]

8 Clinical support

Aims:
➤ National leadership, support, evidence and tools for reconfiguration of pathology services building on the Carter Review.
➤ Targeted service improvement support for applying LEAN processes to pathology services.
➤ Capability development for clinical leadership within pathology services.
➤ Improved interoperability capability for pathology IT services.[1]

9 Productive care

Aims:
➤ Bespoke support and training to increase local capacity and capability to scale up delivery of the Productive series, concentrating on the:
  ➣ Productive Ward.
  ➣ Productive Mental Health Ward.
  ➣ Productive Community Service.
  ➣ Productive Operating Theatre.
➤ Support and tools to enable organisations to reduce their agency costs,

including facilitating the use of useful diagnostic information on variation of staff productivity, and linking workforce to finance and quality measures.[1]

10 Medicines use and procurement

Aims:
- ➤ Clear guidance on the efficient use of medicines in primary care through the National Prescribing Centre and review/expansion of existing Better Care Better Value indicators.
- ➤ Greater transparency and clarity to commissioners and prescribers on the cost of some treatments – for example 'specials'.
- ➤ Best practice tool on medicines management and additional support for primary care trust Prescribing advisers.
- ➤ Additional proposals to improve medicines waste and concordance.[1]

System enablers
11 Primary care contracting and primary care commissioning

Aims:
- ➤ Changes to the GP contract and commissioning framework to support and enable QIPP national workstreams and SHA plans.
- ➤ Support to SHAs to gain maximum value from locally negotiated contracts.[1]

12 Technology and digital vision

Aims:
- ➤ Help to put in place the underpinning technology required for the other national workstreams.
- ➤ Support in the development of regional and local IT strategies.
- ➤ Ensure compatibility and interoperability of IT systems.[1]

SUMMARY
- ➤ 'QIPP' stands for quality, innovation, productivity and prevention and is the response of the NHS to the financial challenge.
- ➤ QIPP works at national, regional and local levels to support clinical teams and NHS organisations to improve the quality of care they deliver while making efficiency savings.

REFERENCE
1 Department of Health. *National Workstreams*. Department of Health; 2010. Available at: www.dh.gov.uk/en/Healthcare/Qualityandproductivity/DH_112316 (accessed 6 December 2010).

CHAPTER 7

Some ideas to save money in the NHS

Disclaimer: Some of the ideas in this chapter are controversial. They should not be taken as the official policy of any organisation that the author is associated with.

POLICY CHANGES
Alcohol and cigarettes
➤ Consider only allowing the sale of cigarettes in pharmacies.
➤ Ban adverts for alcohol and do not allow supermarkets to sell alcohol.
➤ Increase the cost of alcohol.

Pay and pensions
➤ Every full-time equivalent worker in the NHS to get a pay increase of £350 a year for the next three years so lower paid workers benefit more.
➤ Get UK-qualified doctors to take a pay cut of 2% of their salary to acknowledge the cost of training them.
➤ Decrease the pension benefits of all staff earning more than £30 000 a year by 5%.

Autonomy
➤ Allow a greater number of NHS organisations to keep any money not spent at the end of the financial year.

Hours worked
➤ Increase the number of hours junior doctors are allowed to work, from 48 hours up to 55 hours a week.

Advertisements
➤ Allow companies to pay to advertise on the sides of ambulances and on staff uniforms.

Targets
➤ Reduce the four-hour treatment target in A&E.
➤ Allow the increase in waiting times for elective operations.
➤ Decrease the number of patients treated for elective operations in private hospitals paid for by the NHS under the Choice Agenda.

Abroad
➤ NHS to purchase operations to be carried out in foreign countries where this is cheaper but has no worse clinical outcome.
➤ Decrease the cost of NHS Direct by having staff work from call centres abroad.

Tariff
➤ Reduce the price of the tariff that hospitals can charge by 3% a year for the next three years.

BROADER HEALTH
Smoking-related illnesses
➤ Invest in helping people to give up smoking thus reducing the number of smoking-related diseases.
➤ Reduce the number of hospital admissions of those with chronic obstructive pulmonary disease by improving its management in the community.

Cardiovascular disease
➤ Reduce the number of patients developing heart attacks and strokes by improving the management of diseases like hypertension and diabetes.
➤ Ensure there is good access to angioplasty for heart attack cases and thrombolysis for stroke patients.

Prevention
➤ Ensure there is high uptake of immunisations.
➤ Develop innovative ways to reduce the number of children becoming obese.
➤ Have good access to cognitive behavioural therapy for patients with anxiety and depression.
➤ Ensure there is good access to genitourinary services.

CUTTING COSTS
Energy efficiency
➤ Greatly increase the effort towards making the NHS more energy efficient.

Lease
➤ Increase the sale and lease back of NHS property, vehicles and equipment.
➤ Rent out space in hospitals to alternative health practitioners.

Medication
➤ Increase the number of medication reviews to reduce the number of unnecessary mediations being prescribed.
➤ Ensure doctors prescribe cheaper generic drugs rather than branded ones and increase the prescribing of the low cost statins.
➤ Ban doctors meeting with pharmaceutical drug representatives.
➤ Increase the cost of prescription charges by 5% a year above inflation.
➤ Have pharmacists include on the label the actual NHS cost of medication they dispense when it costs the NHS more than £15. This should increase patients' awareness of the cost of their medication and reduce medication wastage.
➤ Encourage consultants caring for older people to review the medication of people in nursing homes, which may result in some medicines being stopped. This will save money and improve patient care.
➤ Greatly decrease the prescribing of 'specials' medication.

Reducing spending
➤ Reduce the spend on IT and on the Department of Health headquarters by 10% a year for the next three years.
➤ Decrease the money spent by the NHS on management consultants by 50%.
➤ Decrease the number of new medical students by 10%.
➤ Reduce by 10% the money spent on units of dental activity, *in vitro* fertilisation (IVF) treatments, personal medical services (PMS) general practices, patient transport, Darzi centres, GP extended hours and independent treatment centres.

DIFFERENT PRACTICES
Avoid duplication
➤ Have greater sharing of resources and functions.
➤ Share back-office functions such as payroll and estates management among NHS organisations.

Threshold of treatment
➤ Change the rationing threshold at which treatment is recommended under the NHS, from £30 000 per quality adjusted life year (QALY) level to £25 000 per QALY.
➤ Increase the present threshold of severity of illness at which patients are able to have cataract operations and joint replacements.
➤ Consider increasing by one week the gestation threshold at which premature babies are treated by special care baby units.

Less variation

➤ Reduce variations in surgical thresholds, in emergency admissions and in outpatient referrals.

➤ Reduce the length of hospital stay.

➤ Increase day-case surgery rates.

➤ Invest money to reduce the number of medically fit patients having delayed discharge from hospital.

➤ Take measures to try to reduce unnecessary readmissions into hospital.

➤ Take measures to reduce the number of appointments not attended by patients.

➤ Reduce unnecessary follow-up appointments.

➤ Shift the treatment of more conditions from hospital to the community; for example, cellulitis, deep vein thrombosis (DVT).

➤ Invest in services that will increase the percentage of palliative care patients dying at home and that reduce the percentage of caesarean section births.

➤ Inform clinicians of the financial cost to the NHS of the investigations they commonly request so that they will think twice before ordering unnecessary tests.

Patient safety

➤ Copy the improvements made to patients' safety brought about by the Institute of Healthcare Improvement in the US.

➤ Train nursing staff in hospitals to identify early those patients who are showing signs of deteriorating.

➤ Reduce the number of hospital-associated infections and patients developing venous thromboembolism in hospitals.

Improved cost-effectiveness

➤ Improve the skill mix so care is provided more cost-effectively.

➤ Pay theatre staff in hospitals for activity rather than for the number of hours worked.

➤ Give further training to junior hospital doctors to increase their awareness of the costs of the medication and the equipment they use.

➤ Provide incentives to front-line staff to deliver more cost-effective care by sharing savings between the hospital and the departments that implement the savings.

Medically unexplained symptoms

➤ Improve training for GPs and hospital doctors so they can better identify patients who have medically unexplained symptoms. These patients have psychological distress that manifests as physical symptoms, often resulting in expensive unnecessary investigations.

THE OLD WAY OF DEALING WITH RESTRICTED FUNDING IN THE NHS

Commissioners:

➤ ensured budgets were not exceeded, even if service quality was greatly affected
➤ reduced spending in health promotion
➤ made cuts where it was politically easier rather than looking objectively at the cost and benefits of where money was spent.

Hospitals, community services and GPs:

➤ thought of their own organisation's best interests rather than what was in the best long-term interests of the NHS in the area
➤ resisted any budget cuts and used patients and media to fight them
➤ resisted new ways of working
➤ blamed the managers.

A BETTER WAY OF DEALING WITH TIGHT FUNDING IN THE NHS

➤ Clinicians explaining to the public why tough decisions are being made.
➤ Greater emphasis on using cost–benefit analysis, e.g. using QALY to make decisions about funding.
➤ Commissioners and providers working more collaboratively to come up with synergistic solutions that save money and/or improve care.
➤ Improving patient safety, which will save money and increase quality of care.
➤ The NHS, local councils and the third sector working together to devise better solutions.
➤ Using good ideas from other sectors.
➤ More emphasis on disease prevention.
➤ Focus on the long-term best interests of patients and the whole system, rather than on the short-term benefits to individuals' own organisations.

FACTORS NEEDED TO BRING ABOUT THIS CULTURAL CHANGE

➤ Leadership that thinks long term and strives for win-win solutions.
➤ Greater trust and openness between commissioners and providers.
➤ Rewards for behaviour that will benefit patients and the NHS in the long term.
➤ The different organisations in the NHS and in social services to work more closely together.

SUMMARY

➤ There are ideas available that could potentially save a large amount of money in the NHS.

➤ It will require courage and trust for some of these ideas to be implemented.

PART 2

Knowledge needed for effective GP commissioning

CHAPTER 8

Assessing local health needs

'Health needs assessment is a systematic method for reviewing the health issues facing a population, leading to agreed priorities and resource allocation that will improve health and reduce inequalities.'[1] It can be the first stage in commissioning, as illustrated in Figure 1.1 (p. 4).

Health Needs Assessment is a recommended public health tool to provide evidence about a population on which to plan services and address health inequalities. It provides an opportunity to engage with specific populations and enables them to contribute to targeted service planning and resource allocation. It also provides an opportunity for cross-sectoral partnership working and developing creative and effective interventions.

Health Needs Assessment offers a vital tool to support national and local priorities.

The benefits of Health Needs Assessment can include:
➤ strengthened community involvement in decision-making
➤ improved team and partnership working
➤ professional development of skills and experience
➤ improved communication with other agencies and the public
➤ better use of resources.[1]

The challenges of Health Needs Assessment are:
➤ working across professional boundaries that prevent power – or information – sharing
➤ developing a shared language between sectors
➤ obtaining commitment from 'the top'
➤ accessing relevant data
➤ accessing the target population
➤ maintaining team impetus and commitment
➤ translating findings into effective action.[1]

Carrying out an effective Health Needs Assessment requires that the related challenges and requirements be considered first; check that:

➤ clear aims and objectives for the project have been identified
➤ there is an established need for the project (e.g. a recent assessment has not already been done)
➤ the right people are involved – this should include:
  ➤ who knows about the issue
  ➤ who cares about the issue
  ➤ who can make change happen
➤ there is sign-up to the project from senior managers and policy makers
➤ a lead coordinator with project management skills can be appointed
➤ access to the target population and their willingness to engage with the project has been established
➤ a committed and skilled project team can be appointed
➤ key stakeholders can be identified
➤ the proposed project team has adequate resources – time, space, equipment, skills and funding – to conduct a good quality Health Needs Assessment.[1]

STEPS IN CARRYING OUT A HEALTH NEEDS ASSESSMENT
Step 1
Getting started
➤ What population?
➤ What are you trying to achieve?
➤ Who needs to be involved?
➤ What resources are required?
➤ What are the risks?

Step 2
Identifying health priorities
➤ Population profiling.
➤ Gathering data.
➤ Perceptions of need.
➤ Identifying and assessing health conditions and determinant factors.

Step 3
Assessing a health priority for action
➤ Choosing health conditions and determinant factors with the most significant size and severity impact.
➤ Determining effective and acceptable interventions and actions.

Step 4
Planning for change
➤ Clarifying aims of intervention.
➤ Action planning.

➤ Monitoring and evaluation strategy.
➤ Risk-management strategy.

Step 5
Moving on/review
➤ Learning from the project.
➤ Measuring impact.
➤ Choosing the next priority.[1]

SUMMARY
➤ Health Needs Assessment is a systematic method for reviewing the health issues facing a population, leading to agreed priorities and resource allocation that will improve health and reduce inequalities.
➤ It can be the first stage in commissioning.

REFERENCE
1 National Institute for Health and Clinical Excellence. *Health Needs Assessment: a practical guide.* London: NIHCE; 2005. Available at: www.nice.org.uk/media/150/35/ Health_Needs_Assessment_A_Practical_Guide.pdf (accessed 8 December 2010). Reproduced with permission.

CHAPTER 9

Budgets

CREATING BUDGETS IN NHS ORGANISATIONS

Creating, monitoring and managing a budget is very important. It helps in the process of allocating resources where they are needed. You need to work out what you are likely to earn and spend in the budget period.

Begin by asking these questions:

1 What is the projected **income** for the budget period?
2 What are the **direct costs** of activity – i.e. costs of materials to supply the service?
3 What are the **fixed costs** or overheads?

You should break down the **fixed costs and overheads** by type, for example:

➤ cost of premises, including rent or mortgage, business rates and service charges
➤ staff costs – e.g. pay, benefits, National Insurance
➤ utilities – e.g. heating, lighting, telephone or internet connection
➤ printing, postage and stationery
➤ vehicle expenses
➤ equipment costs
➤ advertising and promotion
➤ travel and subsistence expenses
➤ legal and professional costs, including insurance.

Your business may have different types of expenses, and you may need to divide the budget by department. Do not forget to add in how much you need to pay yourself, and include an allowance for tax.

Your business plan should help in establishing projected income, cost of activity, fixed costs and overheads, so it would be worthwhile preparing this first.

Once you have figures for income and expenditure, you can work out how much money you are making. You can look at your costs and work out ways to reduce them, as well as seeing if you are likely to have cashflow problems, and giving yourself time to do something about them.

You should stick to your budget as far as possible, but review and revise it as needed.

KEY STEPS IN DRAWING UP A BUDGET

There are a number of key steps you should follow to make sure your budgets and plans are as realistic and useful as possible.

1 Make time for budgeting

If you invest some time in creating a comprehensive and realistic budget, it will be easier to manage and ultimately more effective.

2 Use last year's figures – but only as a guide

Collect historical information on income and costs if they are available – these could give you a good indication of likely future income and costs. It is also essential to consider what your activity plans are and any changes in the competitive environment.

3 Create realistic budgets

Use historical information, your business plan and any changes in operations or priorities to budget for overheads and other fixed costs.

It is useful to work out the relationship between variable costs and activity and then use your activity forecast to project variable costs.

Make sure your budgets contain enough information for you to easily monitor the key drivers of your business such as activity, costs and working capital. Accounting software can help you manage your accounts.

4 Involve the right people

It is best to ask staff with financial responsibilities to provide you with estimates of figures for your budget – for example, activity targets, production costs or specific project control. If you balance their estimates against your own, you will achieve a more realistic budget. This involvement will also give them greater commitment to meeting the budget.

WHAT YOUR BUDGET WILL NEED TO INCLUDE

1 **Projected cashflow**: your cash budget projects your future cash position on a month-by-month basis. Budgeting in this way is vital as it can pinpoint any difficulties you might be having. It should be reviewed at least monthly.
2 **Costs**: typically, your business will have three kinds of costs:
   - ➤ fixed costs – items such as rent, rates, salaries and financing costs
   - ➤ variable costs – including raw materials and overtime

➤ one-off capital costs – for example, purchases of computer equipment or premises

To forecast your costs, it can help to look at last year's records and contact your suppliers for quotes.

3 **Revenues**: activity and income forecasts are typically based on a combination of your activity history and how effective you expect your future efforts to be.

Using your activity and expenditure forecasts, you can prepare projected profits for the next 12 months. This will enable you to analyse your margins and other key ratios such as your return on investment.

SUMMARY

➤ Creating, monitoring and managing a budget is very important. It helps in the process of allocating resources to where they are needed.
➤ You need to work out what you are likely to earn and spend in the budget period.

REFERENCE

Business Link. *Budgets and Business Planning*. Available at www.businesslink.gov.uk/bdotg/action/detail?itemId=1074417146&lang=en&type=RESOURCES (accessed 25 January 2011) ©2009 Crown copyright. Reproduced with the permission of the Controller of HMSO and the Queen's Printer for Scotland.

CHAPTER 10

Business plans

It is essential to have a realistic, working business plan when you are starting up a business.

A business plan is a written document that describes a business, its objectives, its strategies, the market it is in and its financial forecasts. It has many functions, from securing external funding to measuring success within your business.

There are many benefits to creating and managing a realistic business plan. Even if you just use it in-house, it can:

➤ help you spot potential pitfalls before they happen
➤ structure the financial side of your business efficiently
➤ focus your development efforts
➤ work as a measure of your success.[1]

A business plan can be used to secure external funding. This is significant as 'potential investors, including banks, may invest in your idea, work with you or lend you money as a result of the strength of your plan.'[1]

The following people or institutions may request to see your business plan at some stage:

➤ banks
➤ external investors – whether this is a friend, a venture capitalist firm or a business angel
➤ grant providers
➤ anyone interested in buying your business
➤ potential partners.

You should also bear in mind that a business plan is a living document that will need updating and changing as your business grows. Regardless of whether you intend to use your plan internally, or as a document for external people, it should still take an objective and honest look at your business. Failing to do this could mean that you and others have unrealistic expectations of what can be achieved and when.[1]

WHAT THE PLAN SHOULD INCLUDE

Your business plan should provide details of how you are going to develop your business, when you are going to do it, who is going to play a part and how you will manage the finances.

Clarity on these issues is particularly important if you're looking for finance or investment. The process of building your plan will also focus your mind on how your new business will need to operate to give it the best chance of success.

Your plan should include:

➤ **An executive summary** – this is an overview of the business you want to start. It is vital; many lenders and investors make judgments about your business based on this section of the plan alone.

➤ **A short description of the business opportunity** – who you are, what you plan to sell or offer, why and to whom.

➤ **Your marketing and sales strategy** – why you think people will buy what you want to sell and how you plan to sell to them.

➤ **Your management team and personnel** – your credentials and the people you plan to recruit to work with you.

➤ **Your operations** – your premises, facilities, your management information systems and IT.

➤ **Financial forecasts** – this section translates everything you have said in the previous sections into numbers.[1]

SUMMARY

➤ It is essential to have a realistic, working business plan when you are starting up a business.

➤ A business plan is a written document that describes a business, its objectives, strategies, financial forecasts and the market it is in.

REFERENCE

1 Business Link. *Prepare a Business Plan*. Business Link; 2009. Available at: www.business link.gov.uk/bdotg/action/layer?topicId=1073869162 (accessed 8 December 2010). ©2009 Crown copyright. Reproduced with the permission of the Controller of HMSO and the Queen's Printer for Scotland.

CHAPTER 11

Change implementation

REASONS A PERSON MAY RESIST CHANGE

An individual may resist change because they:
➤ do not feel a need to change
➤ do not see what is in it for them to change
➤ do not understand the consequences of not changing
➤ do not agree with the direction of change
➤ do not feel able or competent enough to change
➤ understand the change but fear the consequences of changing
➤ have habits they are used to and will find difficult to break
➤ feel systems do not support the proposed change.

POSSIBLE PERCEIVED LOSSES OF A CHANGE

Losses people perceive may result from change:
➤ job security
➤ psychological comfort/security (the world might become less certain)
➤ purpose or meaning
➤ competence
➤ social connections
➤ future opportunities
➤ power, influence and social status
➤ independence and autonomy.

ORGANISATIONAL DYNAMICS OF CHANGE

➤ Communications deteriorate.
➤ Productivity suffers.
➤ Power/turf struggles occur.
➤ Morale often goes down.
➤ Good people jump ship.

KOTTER'S STEPS FOR ORGANISATIONAL CHANGE

1 Establish a sense of urgency.
2 Create a team with power to bring about change.
3 Develop an appropriate vision and strategy
4 Communicate the vision.
5 Empower action by getting rid of obstacles; changing systems and structures that get in the way; encouraging risk-taking and non-traditional ideas.
6 Generate short-term wins.
7 Consolidate gains and produce more change.
8 Anchor new ways in the culture.

USING INFLUENCE TO BRING ABOUT CHANGE

1 Focus on vital behaviours.
2 Use the six sources of influence:
   i   personal motivation
   ii   personal ability
   iii social motivation
   iv   social ability
   v   structural motivation
   vi   structural ability.

This will be illustrated by two examples of successful change implementation – in Thailand and the US.

Acquired immune deficiency syndrome (AIDS) in Thailand

➤ By 1993 about 1 000 000 Thais were infected with AIDS.
➤ One third of sex workers were HIV positive.
➤ Of the new cases of AIDS in Thailand, 97% were contracted through heterosexual contact with sex workers.
➤ The vital behaviour to be encouraged was 100% condom usage by sex workers.
➤ By the late 1990s new human immunodeficiency virus (HIV) infections had been reduced from 200 000 a year to 25 000 a year.
➤ By 2004 the 100% Condom Use Program had prevented over 5 000 000 cases of HIV.
➤ Personal motivation: an education campaign to teach sex workers that unprotected sex could mean disease, the loss of a job or even death – sex workers had to be encouraged to want to use a condom.
➤ Personal ability: sex workers were trained in negotiation skills, enabling them to handle even the most aggressive customers who demanded sex without a condom.
➤ Social motivation: doctors worked to get the support of opinion leaders in the industry (experienced sex workers and brothel owners) to ensure others would follow their lead.

➤ Social ability: opinion leaders trained the less-experienced workers in how to deal with clients in a way that kept them safe from disease. In addition, doctors ensured that all brothels were simultaneously supportive of the programme. If they were not, customers would have simply gone to the brothels with lax rules.

➤ Structural motivation: the success of the 100% Condom Use Program hinged on the complete compliance of all brothels. Any brothel that employed sex workers found having sex without a condom would first be given a warning, on the next occasion have to pay penalties, and on the third be shut down by the local authorities for non-compliance.

➤ Structural ability: condoms were provided to sex workers by the government free of charge to make condom use easy.

100 000 Lives Campaign, United States

➤ It was estimated that the deaths of 100 000 patients each year in US hospitals were the direct result of a variety of preventable human errors.

➤ In 2005, the Institute for Healthcare Improvement set up a campaign to reduce preventable deaths in hospitals.

➤ Over 3 100 hospitals were involved.

➤ An estimated 122 000 lives were saved within 18 months.

The vital behaviours of the 100 000 Lives Campaign

1 Deploy rapid response teams at the first sign of patient decline.
2 Deliver reliable, evidence-based care for acute myocardial infarction to prevent deaths from heart attacks.
3 Prevent adverse drug events by implementing medication reconciliation.
4 Prevent central line infections by implementing a series of interdependent, scientifically grounded steps.
5 Prevent surgical site infections by reliably delivering the correct perioperative antibiotics at the proper time.
6 Prevent ventilator-associated pneumonia by implementing a series of interdependent, scientifically grounded steps.

Using the six sources of influence in the 100 000 lives campaign

➤ Personal motivation: using real-life examples of patients whose lives could have been saved to increase motivation amongst clinicians and executives.

➤ Personal ability: providing tools and training for hospitals to introduce best practice.

➤ Social motivation: the guilds that are associations and research groups which physicians look to as credible sources help to persuade.

➤ Social ability: some hospitals help to train nearby hospitals on how to bring about the changes needed to save lives.

➤ Structural motivation: changes result in hospitals saving money. The

campaign is aligned with national initiatives. There is widespread media coverage.
➤ Structural ability: free resources and guides to bring about change. Support from mentor hospitals.

SUMMARY

➤ Ideas can change the world, but only when coupled with influence: the ability to change hearts, minds and behaviour.
➤ Several vital behaviours should be focused on to bring about change, as well as all six sources of influence: personal motivation and ability, social motivation and ability, and structural motivation and ability.

REFERENCE

Patterson K, Grenny J, Maxfield D *et al. Influencer: the power to change anything.* New York: McGraw-Hill; 2008.

CHAPTER 12

Commissioning case checklist

Several factors need to be considered when preparing a commissioning case. These include: financial, strategic, clinical, information management and technology (IM&T), estates, procurement, contract, information governance, communications, public health and the provider market.

THE CHECKLIST

	✓
Who is the project lead?	
Who is the clinical lead?	
Who is the finance lead?	
Who is the information lead?	
Who is the IT lead?	
Financial	
Is the activity information reliable and robust?	
Is the financial modelling sound and the planning assumptions appropriate?	
Is the financial information included in the commissioning case correct?	
Is there a sound basis for the costings going forward into procurement?	
Will there be a set cost for service provision or will potential bidders be expected to submit a cost bid for the service?	
Contract and contract management	
What are the contract implications of the commissioning case?	

Strategic	
Do the aims of the commissioning case link with the GP consortia's strategic plan, and general direction for service development?	
Has the projected impact on other services (including secondary care services) been considered and is it appropriate?	
Is there evidence that public and patient involvement has been sought in the development of this commissioning case and is there ongoing patient and public involvement in the case?	
Has an equality impact assessment been undertaken?	
Are there clear success measures that can be monitored sufficiently?	
Clinical	
Does the case demonstrate that the proposed changes to clinical care pathways/ redesigned services are sensible/workable (including details of how pathways will work among providers)?	
Does the case demonstrate that the quality of clinical care provided to patients will be maintained or improved rather than reduced?	
Will the implementation of the commissioning case address the needs of the target population and help to reduce health inequalities in the area?	
Are there any medicines management issues that need to be considered in the commissioning case proposed?	
Procurement	
Is the proposed procurement methodology appropriate?	
Is the proposed timetable and process reasonable?	
What procurement issues need to be considered?	
Information management and technology (IM&T)	
Are IT system implications being addressed?	
Information governance	
Are the information governance implications addressed?	
Communications	
Have communication elements been addressed?	
Are there consultation requirements relating to this project?	

Public health	
Are there public health requirements relating to the project that need to be addressed?	
Estates	
Are there estates implications to the commissioning of this service?	
Provider market	
Has the market been researched?	
Has the market been developed?	
Does the commission case consider all market sectors including voluntary/third sector, private, and so on?	

SUMMARY

➤ Several factors need to be considered when preparing a commissioning case.

➤ These include: financial, strategic, clinical, information management and technology (IM&T), estates, procurement, contract, information governance, communications, public health and the provider market.

CHAPTER 13

Decision-making

A decision is a judgement or choice among two or more alternatives.

Decision-making can be difficult. Almost any decision involves some conflicts or dissatisfaction.

A significant part of decision-making skills is in knowing and practising good decision-making techniques.

RATIONAL APPROACH TO DECISION-MAKING

One of the decision-making techniques is the rational approach. This approach can be summarised in eight steps.

1 Identify the purpose of your decision. What is exactly the problem to be solved?
2 Gather information. What factors does the problem involve?
3 Identify the standards and criteria to judge the alternatives.
4 Brainstorm and list different possible choices. Generate ideas for possible solutions.
5 Evaluate each choice in terms of its consequences. Use your standards and criteria to determine the advantages and disadvantages of each alternative.
6 Determine the best choice.
7 Put the decision into action. Transform your decision into a specific plan of action steps and execute your plan.
8 Evaluate the outcome of your decision and action steps. What lessons can be learnt?

Limitations of the rational approach to decision-making

➤ It may be difficult to find sufficient relevant information to make a rational decision.
➤ There may be competing or conflicting interests and objectives.
➤ It may be time-consuming to determine the best choice.
➤ It may be expensive to determine the best choice.

Alternatives to the rational approach to decision-making

➤ Modified rational approach: follow the basic line of the rational approach but not so rigorously.

➤ Less-than-ideal approach: consider choosing an option that falls short of, but is as close as possible to your ideal.

➤ Intuitive but honest approach: make your choice intuitively, but be honest with yourself and spell out the real reasons why you chose that alternative.

➤ Negative approach: look for reasons to reject options until you are left with the most preferable of the remaining options.

➤ Changing circumstances approach: consider what will happen if circumstances were changed and choose the option that remains best in these changed circumstances.

BRAINSTORMING

This is a group creativity technique designed to generate a large number of ideas for the solution of a problem.

There are four basic rules in brainstorming. These are intended to reduce social inhibitions among group members, stimulate idea generation, and increase overall creativity of the group.

1 **Focus on quantity**.

This rule is a means of enhancing divergent thinking using the principal quantity will breed quality.

The assumption is that the greater the number of ideas generated, the greater the chance of finding a radical and effective solution which will solve the problem.

2 **Withhold criticism**.

In brainstorming, criticism of ideas generated should be postponed.

Participants should focus on extending or adding to ideas, reserving criticism for a later stage.

By suspending judgment, participants will not be scared to generate unusual ideas.

3 **Welcome unusual ideas**.

To get a good and long list of ideas, unusual ideas are welcomed.

They can be generated by looking from new perspectives and suspending assumptions.

These new ways of thinking may provide better solutions.

4 **Combine and improve ideas**.

Good ideas may be combined to form a single better idea.

SUMMARY

➤ The rational approach to decision-making is to identify the purpose of your decision, gather information, identify the standards and criteria to judge the alternatives, brainstorm and list different possible choices, evaluate each choice in terms of its consequences, determine the best choice, put the decision into action and finally evaluate the outcome of your decision.

➤ The rules of brainstorming are: focus on quantity, withhold criticism, welcome unusual ideas, and combine and improve ideas.

CHAPTER 14

Delegation

Delegation is about entrusting others with appropriate responsibility and authority for performing certain activities or accomplishing specific goals.

BENEFITS OF DELEGATION

Delegation:

➤ motivates the people to whom work is delegated to by giving them more challenging work
➤ frees up the time of the person delegating so they can do their most important tasks
➤ reduces the stress level of both the person delegating and the person being delegated to
➤ encourages the delegator to prioritise their work
➤ helps the delegator to assess the potential of the people who work for them
➤ contributes to succession planning by exposing people to other levels of work
➤ serves as a development tool by increasing the range of skills in a team.

THE STEPS OF SUCCESSFUL DELEGATION

1 **Choose an appropriate task**: check that the task is one suitable to be delegated and not just an unpleasant task that you don't want to do yourself.
2 **Select the appropriate person to delegate to**: consider the reasons for delegating and the benefits to you and the person you are delegating to. Ensure the person you are delegating to is capable of doing the task.
3 **Explain the task**: explain to the person accepting the task what is required, its importance, where it fits in the overall picture and why you are delegating it. Explain what must be achieved. Ensure the person being delegated to understands and ask them for their ideas and suggestions.
4 **Supply the necessary resources**: agree what resources are required to complete the task, for example, money, people, and so on.
5 **Agree deadlines**: agree when the task should be finished and when

progress will be reviewed (failing to agree in advance on a review time will cause this monitoring to seem like interference or lack of trust).

6 **Support and communicate**: inform your peers and/or your own boss, if it is relevant, of the new responsibilities of the person you are delegating to. Warn the person you are delegating to about any potential pitfalls, such as office politics.

7 **Feedback on results**: let the person know how well they completed the task and give them credit for any success, but you should absorb the consequences of any failure.

LEVELS OF AUTHORITY

It is also important to make sure that the person you are delegating to has the right amount of authority. There are eight levels:

1 The delegatee gets all the facts then the delegator makes the decision.
2 The delegatee report the pros and cons of alternatives and the delegator makes the decision.
3 The delegatee recommends a particular action and delegator makes the final decision.
4 The delegatee decides the action and waits for the approval of the delagator.
5 The delegatee decides the action and acts unless the delegator says not to.
6 The delegatee acts and tells the delegator what happened.
7 The delegatee acts and only tells the delegator if it is unsuccessful.
8 The delegate acts and no report is necessary.

SUMMARY

➤ Delegation is about entrusting others with appropriate responsibility and authority for performing certain activities or accomplishing specific goals.

➤ It has several benefits including motivating the people delegated to and freeing up the person delegating to do their most important tasks.

➤ It involves choosing an appropriate task, selecting an appropriate person to delegate to, explaining the task, supplying the necessary resources, agreeing on deadlines, supporting and communicating, and giving feedback on the results.

CHAPTER 15

Emails

QUESTIONS TO CONSIDER BEFORE SENDING AN EMAIL

➤ What am I trying to achieve by sending this email?
➤ Would a phone call or a face-to-face meeting be more appropriate than an email?
➤ Am I sending the email to too many people?
➤ How can I make this email short, concise and action focused?
➤ Am I sending an email that I will later regret sending?
➤ How can I make the subject line clear and meaningful?

LANGUAGE

➤ The email should be brief and to the point.
➤ The language, style and tone used should be suitable for the target audience and their level of understanding of the subject.
➤ Abbreviations should be kept to a minimum.
➤ A spell check facility should be used and the message proofread before sending.

FORMATTING

➤ Use paragraphs, bullet points and numbering to structure the email.
➤ Only use bold and underlining to emphasise key points.
➤ Use an electronic signature with contact information.

ATTACHMENTS

➤ Try to avoid sending email attachments when the recipient has access to the same server and shared files – use web links instead.
➤ Reduce the size of documents by compressing them where possible.

THINGS TO AVOID

➤ Sending an email with no subject.
➤ Sending an email when you are very angry.
➤ Marking an email as urgent in anything more than a very small percentage of the emails you send.
➤ Writing a very long email with big paragraphs.
➤ Lots of spelling mistakes.
➤ Replying to all recipients unless it is absolutely necessary.
➤ Sending unnecessary emails.

DEALING WITH EMAILS YOU RECEIVE

➤ Schedule time to deal with emails as part of your working week.
➤ Reply to an email immediately if it will take less than two minutes.
➤ Delete those emails that can be deleted.
➤ Delegate those emails that can be delegated.
➤ Put emails that cannot be dealt with now in a to-do folder.

SUMMARY

➤ Consider what you are hoping to achieve before sending an email.
➤ Try to send emails that are short, concise and action focused.
➤ Have a plan to deal with the emails you receive.

CHAPTER 16

Ethics

MEDICAL ETHICS
➤ Medical ethics is the study of moral values and judgements as they apply to medicine.
➤ Medical ethics has a role to play in the decision-making about which treatments the NHS funds and which it does not.
➤ There is public interest and public scrutiny over ethical decisions made by the NHS.

VALUES APPLIED TO MEDICAL ETHICS
➤ Beneficence – a practitioner should act in the best interest of the patient.
➤ Non-maleficence – 'first, do no harm'.
➤ Autonomy – the patient has the right to refuse or choose their treatment.
➤ Justice – concerns the distribution of scarce health resources, and the decision of who gets what treatment (fairness and equality).
➤ Dignity – the patient has the right to dignity.
➤ Truthfulness and honesty and the concept of informed consent.

How to decide the right action in a particular situation
➤ Values such as these do not give answers as to how to handle a particular situation, but provide a useful framework for understanding conflicts.
➤ When moral values are in conflict, the result may be an ethical dilemma.
➤ The General Medical Council (GMC) provides guidance in the form of its Good Medical Practice and Management for Doctors documents.

GOOD MEDICAL PRACTICE: GUIDANCE FOR DOCTORS (2006)[1]
The duties of a doctor
Below are some parts of this guidance from the GMC. The full guidance is available online.[1]

Patients must be able to trust doctors with their lives and health. To justify that trust you must show respect for human life and you must:

➤ Make the care of your patient your first concern.
➤ Protect and promote the health of patients and the public.
➤ Provide a good standard of practice and care:
   ➣ keep your professional knowledge and skills up to date
   ➣ recognise and work within the limits of your competence
   ➣ work with colleagues in the ways that best serve patients' interests.
➤ Work in partnership with patients:
   ➣ listen to patients and respond to their concerns and preferences
   ➣ give patients the information they want or need in a way they can understand
   ➣ respect patients' right to reach decisions with you about their treatment and care
   ➣ support patients in caring for themselves to improve and maintain their health.
➤ Treat patients as individuals and respect their dignity:
   ➣ treat patients politely and considerately
   ➣ respect patients' right to confidentiality.
➤ Be honest and open and act with integrity:
   ➣ act without delay if you have good reason to believe that you or a colleague may be putting patients at risk
   ➣ never discriminate unfairly against patients or colleagues
   ➣ never abuse your patients' trust in you or the public's trust in the profession.
➤ You are personally accountable for your professional practice and must always be prepared to justify your decisions and actions.[1]

MANAGEMENT FOR DOCTORS: GUIDANCE FOR DOCTORS (2009)[2]

Below are some parts of this guidance from the GMC. The full guidance is available online.[2]

4 You continue to have a duty of care for the safety and well-being of patients when you work as a manager. You remain accountable to the GMC for your decisions and actions even when a non-doctor could perform your management role.

5 *Good Medical Practice* sets out the fundamental principles that should underpin the practice of all doctors.

8 The Committee on Standards in Public Life (the Nolan Committee) set out seven principles for the conduct of holders of public office. The principles have been widely accepted as applicable in areas far wider than those for which they were initially drawn up, and they offer a useful set of principles for doctors who manage.

9 The seven principles are:

➢ selflessness
➢ integrity
➢ objectivity
➢ accountability
➢ openness
➢ honesty
➢ leadership.

10 All practising doctors use resources and play a role in setting priorities, developing policies and making other management decisions. All doctors have an obligation therefore to work with both medical and non-medical managers in a productive way for the benefit of patients and the public.

Providing a good standard of management practice

12 It is not possible to set out all the roles doctors take on as managers. If your role involves responsibilities covered in this booklet, you should do your best to make sure that:

➢ systems are in place to enable high-quality medical services to be provided
➢ care is provided and supervised only by staff who have the appropriate skills (including communication skills), experience, training and qualifications
➢ significant risks to patients, staff and the health of the wider community are identified, assessed and addressed to minimise risk, and that they are reported in line with local and national procedures
➢ the people you manage (both doctors and other professionals) are aware of and follow the guidance issued by relevant professional and regulatory bodies, and that they are able to fulfil their professional duties so that standards of practice and care are maintained and improved
➢ systems are in place to identify the educational and training needs of students and staff, including locums, so that the best use is made of the time and resources available for keeping knowledge and skills up to date
➢ all decisions, working practices and the working environment are lawful, with particular regard to the law on employment, equal opportunities and health and safety
➢ information and policies on clinical effectiveness and clinical governance are publicised and implemented effectively.

Competencies and standards that define a good manager

17 As an effective manager, you should be able to:

➢ lead a team effectively
➢ identify and set objectives

> communicate clearly
> manage resources and plan work to achieve maximum benefits, both day to day and in the longer term
> make sound decisions in difficult situations
> know when to seek help and do so when appropriate
> offer help to those you manage, when they need it
> demonstrate leadership qualities through your own example
> manage projects
> manage change
> delegate appropriately – to empower others, to improve services and to develop the skills of the people you manage – without giving up your own responsibilities
> consider and act upon constructive feedback from colleagues.

18 As an effective manager, you need a sound working knowledge of the:
> main clinical and other issues relevant to those you manage
> key skills and contributions of other health professionals
> roles and policies of local agencies involved in healthcare
> needs of patients, carers and colleagues
> use and application of information and information technology
> nature of clinical and other risks
> limits of what is affordable and achievable
> principles of change management
> culture of the organisations in which you work
> structure and lines of accountability in the organisation in which you work
> principles of good employment practice and effective people management.

Responsibilities, conflict and accountability

20 Whether you have a management role or not, your primary duty is to your patients. Their care and safety must be your first concern. You also have a duty to the health of the wider community, your profession, your colleagues, and the organisation in which you work.

21 Management involves making judgements about competing demands on available resources. If managerial concerns conflict with your primary duty to the extent that you are concerned for the safety or well-being of your patients, you should declare the conflict, seek colleagues' advice, and raise your concerns formally with senior management and external professional bodies as appropriate.

22 At times you may not have the resources to provide the best treatment or care that all your patients need. At such times your decisions should be based on sound research information on efficiency and efficacy, and in line with your duties to protect life and health, to respect patients' autonomy and to treat justly.

Leading teams

50 When leading a team you should:
  - Respect the skills and contributions of your colleagues; you must not make unfounded criticisms of colleagues, which can undermine patients' trust in the care provided.
  - Make sure that colleagues understand the professional status and specialty of all team members, their roles and responsibilities in the team, and who is responsible for each aspect of patient care.
  - Make sure that staff are clear about their individual and team objectives, their personal and collective responsibilities for patient and public safety, and for openly and honestly recording and discussing problems.
  - Communicate effectively with colleagues within and outside the team; you should make sure that arrangements are in place for relevant information to be passed on to the team promptly.
  - Make sure that all team members have an opportunity to contribute to discussions and that they understand and accept the decisions taken.
  - Encourage team members to cooperate and communicate effectively with each other.
  - Make sure that each patient's care is properly coordinated and managed, and that patients are given information about whom to contact if they have questions or concerns; this is particularly important when patient care is shared between teams.
  - Set up and maintain systems to identify and manage risks in the team's area of responsibility.
  - Monitor and regularly review the team's performance and take steps to correct deficiencies and improve quality.
  - Deal openly and supportively with problems in the conduct, performance or health of team members through effective and well-publicised procedures.
  - Make sure that your team and the organisation have the opportunity to learn from mistakes.

Financial and commercial dealings

54 You must be open and honest in any financial and commercial dealings you are responsible for. You must make sure that you and those you manage are competent and have the necessary training or advice for any financial work you take on.

55 You must declare any interests you have that could influence or be seen to influence your judgement in any financial or commercial dealings you are responsible for. In particular, you must not allow your interests to influence:
  - the treatment of patients
  - purchases from funds for which you are responsible

➤ the terms or awarding of contracts
➤ the conduct of research.

56 You should make sure there are adequate systems in place to monitor financial and management information and that you and those you manage make full use of them. This includes awarding contracts and managing waiting lists and service plans.

57 You must make sure that the funds you manage are used for the purposes they were intended for and are clearly and properly accounted for. You should also make sure that appropriate professional services, including audit, are commissioned when necessary.[2]

SUMMARY

➤ Medical ethics can help the NHS when it has to decide which treatments should be funded.

➤ The GMC provides guidance for doctors in management, which has to be followed.

REFERENCES

1 General Medical Council. *Good Medical Practice: guidance for doctors*. London: General Medical Council; 2009. Available at: www.gmc-uk.org/static/documents/content/GMP_0910.pdf (accessed 9 December 2010).

2 General Medical Council. *Management for Doctors: guidance for doctors*. London: General Medical Council; 2006. Available at: www.gmc-uk.org/Management_for_doctors_2006.pdf_27493833.pdf (accessed 9 December 2010).

CHAPTER 17

Financial accounts

Financial accounts are a historical record of a business' performance over a past period – usually one year – for the benefit of external users such as shareholders, employees, suppliers, bankers and authorities.

Financial accounts normally include the following elements.[1]

PROFIT AND LOSS ACCOUNT

This measures a business' performance over a given period of time, usually one year.

It compares the income of the business against the cost of goods or services and expenses incurred in earning that revenue.[1]

BALANCE SHEET

This is a snapshot of a business' assets (what is owns or is owed to it) and its liabilities (what it owes) on a particular day – e.g. the last day of your financial year.[1]

Balance sheets show:
➤ fixed assets – long-term possessions
➤ current assets – short-term possessions
➤ current liabilities – what the business owes and must repay in the short term
➤ long-term liabilities – including owner's or shareholders' capital.

The balance sheet is so called because there is a debit entry and a credit entry for everything (but one entry may be to the profit and loss account), so the total value of the assets is always the same value as the total of the liabilities.

Fixed assets include:
➤ tangible assets – e.g. buildings, land, machinery, computers, fixtures and fittings – shown at their depreciated or resale value where appropriate
➤ intangible assets – e.g. goodwill, intellectual property rights (such as patents, trademarks and website domain names) and long-term investments.

Current assets are short-term assets whose value can fluctuate from day to day and can include:
➤ stock
➤ work in progress
➤ money owed by customers
➤ cash in hand or at the bank
➤ short-term investments
➤ pre-payments – e.g. advance rents.[2]

Current liabilities are amounts owing and due within one year. These include:
➤ money owed to suppliers
➤ short-term loans, overdrafts or other finance
➤ taxes due within the year – VAT [value added tax], PAYE [pay as you earn] and National Insurance.[2]

Long-term liabilities include:
➤ creditors due after one year.
➤ capital and reserves – share capital and retained profits, after dividends (if your business is a limited company), or proprietor's capital invested.[2]

CASHFLOW STATEMENT
➤ This shows how the business has generated and disposed of cash and liquid funds during the period under review.[1]

SUMMARY
➤ Financial accounts are a historical record of a business' performance over a past period.
➤ They include the profit and loss account, balance sheet and cashflow statement.

REFERENCES
1 Business Link. *Financial and Management Accounts: the basics.* Business Link; 2009. Available at: www.businesslink.gov.uk/bdotg/action/detail?itemId=1073791253& type=RESOURCES (accessed 9 December 2010). ©2009 Crown copyright. Reproduced with the permission of the Controller of HMSO and the Queen's Printer for Scotland.
2 Business Link. *Balance Sheets: the basics.* Business Link; 2009. Available at: www. businesslink.gov.uk/bdotg/action/detail?itemId=1074499496&type=RESOURCES (accessed 9 December 2010). ©2009 Crown copyright. Reproduced with the permission of the Controller of HMSO and the Queen's Printer for Scotland.

CHAPTER 18

Integration

IMPROVING THE INTERFACE BETWEEN PRIMARY AND SECONDARY CARE

➤ Each part of the system tends to focus on its own tasks and resources.
➤ The roles of improving the quality of interaction, cooperation and communication across the interface is not seen as any one person's or organisation's particular responsibility.

PATIENTS' VIEWS ON CARE ACROSS THE PRIMARY/ SECONDARY INTERFACE

Preston *et al.* interviewed patients who:
➤ wanted understandable and consistent information, presented in an honest and sympathetic way
➤ wanted continuity of care
➤ wanted to make progress in getting their problem sorted
➤ did not want impersonal care organised according to the routines of staff/organisation.[1]

EUROPEAN WORKING PARTY ON QUALITY IN FAMILY PRACTICE (2001)

➤ The working party identified 10 areas to improve on in the interface between primary and secondary care:
  1 leadership
  2 shared care approaches
  3 consensus on task division
  4 mutual guidelines
  5 patient perspective
  6 informatics
  7 education
  8 team building

9 monitoring quality in clinical work
10 cost-effectiveness.

Some recommendations of the working party:
➤ local management structures designed to encourage care across boundaries
➤ local GPs and specialists establish local guidelines together
➤ patient perspective included in guidelines
➤ effort spent in improving team working
➤ have easy access to information about clinical guidelines
➤ sharing of accurate and timely information between clinicians
➤ joint education courses for specialists and GPs
➤ doing audits, patient surveys and monitoring outcomes and easy access to information about quality of services.

RECENT TECHNICAL IMPROVEMENTS IN THE PRIMARY/ SECONDARY INTERFACE

1 Patient Pathways, NHS Scotland.
2 Information to GPs from the North East Essex clinical website.
3 Software connecting hospital pathology results to GP records.
4 Software allowing other clinicians to access GP records.

1 Patient Pathways, NHS Scotland

National Patient Pathways: www.pathways.scot.nhs.uk
➤ These are evidence-based pathways written by teams from primary and secondary care.
➤ They can form the basis of local guidelines to GPs on:
  ➢ referral criteria for consultants
  ➢ alternative referral to allied health professionals/specialist nurses
  ➢ follow-up options
  ➢ diagnostic tests
  ➢ management tips.
➤ They can also act as an educational tool and provide sources of patient information.

2 NHS North East Essex Clinical Website

www.clinical.northeastessexpct.nhs.uk/Clinical%20Information.htm
  The site contains information such as:
➤ guidelines both local and national
➤ a list of services and how to refer to them
➤ referral criteria and referral forms
➤ patient information leaflets
➤ tools to help in diagnosis.

3 Software connecting hospital pathology results to GP records

The software which is called ICE:

➤ allows GPs to access results of investigations ordered by local hospital or GP, such as blood tests, microbiological investigations and radiological investigations

➤ prevents unnecessary duplication of blood tests

➤ makes available hospital discharge letters and, in the future, hospital outpatients letters.

4 Software from one of the major GP software companies

EMIS web software will:

➤ allow clinicians outside general practice to access a patient's GP medical record

➤ offer access to a series of separate records for the same patient, e.g. GP record, district nursing record, any information supplied by the patient, and so on.

➤ allow data to be shared and viewed with explicit patient consent and according to local data-sharing agreements

➤ allow out of hours or urgent care clinicians to access a patient's GP medical record.

SUMMARY

➤ IT will improve the interface between primary and secondary care over the next few years.

➤ The biggest advance, however, will be improved cooperation, trust and communication and a move to a more long-term, win-win relationship between the two sectors.

REFERENCE

1 Preston C, Cheater F, Baker R *et al*. Left in limbo: patients' views on care across the primary/secondary interface. *Qual Health Care*. 1999; 8: 16–21.

CHAPTER 19

Key terms

The majority of these definitions are taken from the Improving and Integrating Respiratory Services in the NHS (IMPRESS) website.[1]

BENCHMARKING (SOCIAL CARE)

This is a method for councils to work out how well they are doing by comparing their performance with other similar councils, and with performance indicators (PIs). It is also used by PCTs, and various information sources such as the NHS Information Centre now to enable statutory organisations to select benchmarking groups and national data sets in health and social care to compare performance.

CARE PATHWAY

To improve the person-centred nature of care, commissioners and service planners now try to understand how patients experience their care from prevention, to diagnosis and assessment, to treatment and, where appropriate, to palliative care. This normally involves mapping the journey and the experience using a range of techniques with patients, clinicians and managers. They describe this journey as a care pathway. Their aim is to improve the flow of patients along this pathway by reducing inefficiencies and improving reliability.

CHOICE

Since January 2006 in England, patients were offered the choice of at least four hospitals and a booked appointment when they need a referral for elective care. Recently, patients have been able to choose any healthcare provider that meets NHS standards – that is, it may be an independent/private sector provider – and can provide care within the price the NHS is prepared to pay.[1]

CQUIN
Commissioning for Quality and Innovation is a payment framework that functions as a local bonus scheme whereby trusts and other providers are paid additional funding if they reach targets agreed with local commissioners. The CQUIN targets are in the domains of safety, effectiveness, user experience and innovation.

ELECTIVE CARE
Planned care for a pre-existing illness or condition.

ENGAGEMENT
The process of involving others at an individual and collective level. It starts with information, then feedback, then influence.

HEALTHCARE RESOURCE GROUPS (HRGS)
A way of grouping the hospital treatment of patients by case mix to allow analysis of the appropriateness, efficiency and effectiveness of care. Each group contains cases that are clinically similar and will consume similar quantities of healthcare resources. There are, for example, a number of codes which would naturally map to the HRG 'COPD', e.g. emphysema; chronic obstructive pulmonary disease, unspecified; chronic obstructive pulmonary disease with acute exacerbation, etc. These should all represent a similar demand on resources.

INDEPENDENT SECTOR (IS)
An umbrella term for all non-NHS bodies delivering healthcare, including a wide range of private companies and voluntary organisations.

INTEGRATED CARE ORGANISATIONS (ICOS)
These form part of the Next Stage Review and are seen as a means of achieving improved coordination of care, delivering better services between secondary, primary and social care, and providing improved overall care for patients more economically. Core features include primary care involvement. They may be disease-specific or generic services. Social care is not compulsory. Indeed, the term 'integrated care' can be used, as it is for IMPRESS, to mean care crossing primary, community and secondary care boundaries, but it can also mean integration between health and social care.

INTERMEDIATE CARE
Also known as step-up, step-down and transitional care – this is care out of hospital for people who are medically stable but still need temporary care in a community bed or home care for recovery and rehabilitation. Commissioners

are increasing their investment in such services in order to provide care closer to home, to reduce avoidable admissions and excess lengths of stay. The services are often nurse-led but there needs to be clear agreement about medical responsibility.

JOINT STRATEGIC NEEDS ASSESSMENT (JSNA)

A JSNA is the means by which primary care trusts and local authorities will describe the future health, care and well-being needs of local populations, and the strategic direction of service delivery to meet those needs. JSNAs form the basis of a new duty to cooperate for PCTs and local authorities that is contained in the Local Government and Public Involvement in Health Bill. JSNAs take account of data and information on inequalities between the differing, and overlapping, communities in local areas and support the meeting of statutory requirements in relation to equality audits.

LOCAL AREA AGREEMENT (LAA)

A three-year agreement setting out the priorities for funding and delivery for a local area in certain policy fields as agreed between central government (represented by the Government Office), and a local area, represented by the local authority and local strategic partnership and other partners at the local level. It sets out the 'deal' between central government and local authorities and their partners to improve the quality of life for local people.

OPERATING FRAMEWORK

For the NHS in England this is produced annually to give NHS organisations the Department of Health's priorities and planning guidance.

PATIENT-REPORTED OUTCOME MEASURES (PROMS)

These are short, self-completed questionnaires which measure the patient's health status or health-related quality of life at a single point in time and can be repeated to derive a measure of the impact of healthcare interventions.

PAYMENT BY RESULTS (PBR)

How acute providers in England are paid. There is a national fixed tariff for emergency care, elective inpatients, day cases and outpatients bought by NHS commissioners. It does not yet include community services. The important principle is that only work done and recorded using appropriate coding is paid for.

PROVIDER

A generic term for an organisation that delivers a healthcare or care service.

REFERENCE COSTS

These are used in calculating the tariff. They are average costs for providing a defined service in a given financial year. They cover a broad range of NHS treatments and clinical procedures and have been collected since 1998.

SECONDARY CARE

The collective term for services to which a person is referred after the first point of contact. Usually this refers to hospitals in the NHS offering specialised medical services and care (outpatient and inpatient services).

SELF-CARE

Individuals taking responsibility for their own health and well-being and to care for themselves. This includes taking exercise, eating well, taking action to prevent illness and accidents, the better use of medicines, treatment of minor ailments, and better care of long-term conditions.

SERVICE LEVEL AGREEMENT (SLA)

The agreement between the commissioner and provider is in two parts. The SLA, or contract, and the service specification. The SLA is a formal written agreement and is a standard document written by the Department of Health.

SERVICE SPECIFICATION

This is part of the SLA and specifies in detail how and what services will be provided, including the quality standards that the service should maintain. It is useful to read the service specification because it also explains how the services will be monitored.

SOCIAL ENTERPRISE

Businesses with primarily social objectives. Their surpluses are reinvested principally in the business or the community rather than to shareholders. A number of provider services from PCTs are exploring the social enterprise model as a way of setting themselves up apart from the PCT, supported by the Department of Health.

SPELL

The continuous period from a patient's admission to discharge from a hospital, even if they are under the care of several consultants during that time – hence different from the previously used Finished Consultant Episode (FCE).

SECONDARY USES SERVICE (SUS)

The primary use of data in the NHS is to support patient care. Its use for planning and commissioning is a secondary use, hence the name. SUS is the single data warehouse and analysis centre created by the NHS Information Centre pooling Hospital Episode Statistics (HES) and other data collected by providers of NHS care to meet the dataset requirements of NHS commissioners. Every secondary care provider in England has to send a set of standard data files (Commissioning Data Sets) to the SUS system. These files contain details of all the care they have provided, including that covered by Payment by Result (PbR).

TARIFF

This is the amount that a commissioner will pay for a particular package of care including outpatient appointments, spells and procedures. Commissioners now only pay for work that has been done, according to the nationally set tariff with minor local differences when a market forces factor is applied. The tariff is based on a reference cost created from a large retrospective analysis of average costs incurred by NHS hospital providers.

THIRD SECTOR

The full range of non-public, not-for-profit organisations that are non-governmental and 'value driven'; that is, motivated by the desire to further social, environmental or cultural objectives rather than to make a profit.

TOTAL PLACE

Total Place was launched in the 2009 Budget as an initiative led by the Treasury to look at how a 'whole area' approach to public services can lead to better services at less cost. It seeks to identify and avoid overlap and duplication between organisations, look at freedoms from central control, and taking away ring-fences and bureaucratic burdens.

TRIMPOINTS

These are the length of stay up to which an individual tariff applies. They are spell – not FCE – based and, like the tariff itself, are calculated from a large retrospective analysis of average length of stays for particular HRGs. There are separate trimpoints for elective and non-elective activity and some non-elective activity is divided into subgroups according to complexity but this is not very sophisticated at present.

TUPE

Transfer of Undertakings (Protection of Employment) Regulations (2006). Designed to protect the rights of employees in a transfer situation (when a new employer takes over).[1]

URGENT CARE

The Department of Health describes this as primary care for people who would otherwise attend A&E departments or who want a drop-in service. Urgent care centres tend to be either services adjacent to A&E departments that provide an option for patients without an appointment who have a minor injury or illness, or services that expand the range of services currently provided by walk-in centres, minor injury units or community hospitals.

VARIATION

This is the focus for many commissioners. Two broad definitions of variation are usually considered: avoidable variation ('unwarranted') by healthcare professionals and variation ('warranted') due to differences between patients that need to be considered by professionals when offering personalised care. There is much work in the NHS looking at both sides – how to reduce variation applying reliability science, as well as how to empower patients to achieve shared decisions with their healthcare professionals.

VIRTUAL WARDS

These are part of an approach to reducing admissions using the Combined Predictive Risk Model to identify people at risk of admission and to provide a team approach to managing their care in the community.

VOLUNTARY AND COMMUNITY SECTOR

An umbrella term referring to registered charities as well as non-charitable non-profit organisations, associations, self-help groups and community groups, for public or community benefit.[1]

REFERENCE

1 Improving and Integrating Respiratory Services in the NHS (IMPRESS). *Jargon Buster A–Z.* IMPRESS; 2010. Available at: www.impressresp.com/JargonBusterAZ.aspx (accessed 10 December 2010).

CHAPTER 20

Long-term conditions management

Long-term conditions management is based on categorizing care according to risk stratification.[1]

Deciding the right approach
It is important to have the information and knowledge to be able to carry out a risk-stratification on local populations to identify those who are most at risk.

Level 3
As people develop more than one chronic condition (co-morbidities), their care becomes disproportionately more complex and difficult for them, or the health and social care system, to manage. This calls for case management – with a key worker (often a nurse) actively managing and joining up care for these people.

Level 2
Disease/care management, in which multidisciplinary teams provide high-quality evidence-based care to patients, is appropriate for the majority of people at this level. This means proactive management of care, following agreed protocols and pathways for managing specific diseases. It is underpinned by good information systems – patient registries, care planning, shared electronic health records.

Level 1
With the right support many people can learn to be an active participant in their own care, living with and managing their conditions. This can help them to prevent complications, slow down deterioration and avoid getting further conditions. The majority of people with chronic conditions fall into this category – so even small improvements can have a huge impact.

Level 3
Highly complex patients
Case management

Level 2
High-risk patients
Case management

Level 1
70%–80% of a Chronic Care Management population

Health Promotion

FIGURE 20.1 Chronic disease management: population management. Reproduced with permission.[1]

➤ **Level 1** is for patients who can manage their own care and care for themselves, as long as they receive education and support from primary care.

➤ **Level 2** care management is where there is a structured, protocol-driven approach to care.

➤ **Level 3** case management is where a patient needs help to coordinate their care if they are to avoid a succession of unplanned interventions. This is where community matrons and others have been focused.

Figure 20.2 from Castlefields Health Centre develops the model showing how self-care and self-management happens at all levels, and how well they are enabled is probably the most important factor in determining how patients use services.[1]

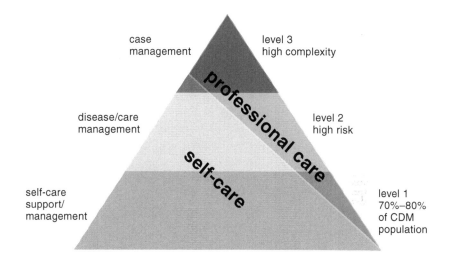

FIGURE 20.2 Chronic disease management and shared case. Source: Castlefields Health Centre. Reproduced with permission.

SUMMARY

➤ Long-term conditions management is based on categorising care according to risk stratification.

REFERENCE

1 Improving and Integrating Respiratory Services in the NHS (IMPRESS). Long term conditions (LTC) management. *Jargon Buster A–Z*. IMPRESS; 2010. Available at: www.impressresp.com/JargonBuster/JargonBusterAZ/tabid/63/FilterID/51/Default. aspx (accessed 10 December 2010).

CHAPTER 21

Management theories

This chapter gives a brief introduction to some useful management theories.

JOB SPECIALISATION AND THE DIVISION OF LABOUR (ADAM SMITH, 18th CENTURY)

Adam Smith (18th century economist):
➤ observed that firms manufactured pins in one of two different ways:
  ➣ craft-style – each worker did all steps
  ➣ production – each worker specialised in one step
➤ realised that job specialisation resulted in much higher efficiency and productivity
➤ breaking down the total job allowed for the division of labour in which workers became very skilled at their specific tasks.

SCIENTIFIC MANAGEMENT (FREDERICK W TAYLOR, 1880s AND 1890s)

➤ Replace rule-of-thumb work methods with scientifically devised methods.
➤ Scientifically select, train, teach and develop each worker instead of leaving them to train themselves.
➤ Provide detailed instructions and supervision of each worker.
➤ Piece-rate pay.

PRINCIPLES OF MANAGEMENT (HENRI FAYOL, 1916)

➤ Division of labour allows for job specialisation: Fayol noted jobs can have too much specialisation leading to poor quality and worker dissatisfaction.
➤ Authority and responsibility: Fayol included both formal and informal authority resulting from special expertise.
➤ Discipline: obedient, applied, respectful employees are necessary for the organisation to function.

➤ Unity of command: employees should have only one boss.
➤ Unity of direction: a single plan of action to guide the organisation.
➤ Subordination of individual interest to the common interest: the interest of the organisation takes precedence over that of the individual employee.
➤ Remuneration of personnel: an equitable uniform payment system that motivates will contribute to organisational success.
➤ Centralisation: the degree to which authority rests at the top of the organisation.
➤ Line of authority: a clear chain of command from the top to the bottom of the firm.
➤ Order: the arrangement of employees where they will be of the most value to the organisation and to provide career opportunities.
➤ Equity: the provision of justice and the fair and impartial treatment of all employees.
➤ Stability of tenure of personnel: long-term employment is important for the development of skills that improve the organisation's performance.
➤ Initiative: the fostering of creativity and innovation by encouraging employees to act on their own.
➤ *Esprit de corps*: comradeship and shared enthusiasm foster devotion to the common cause (organisation).

FIVE PRINCIPLES OF BUREAUCRACY (MAX WEBER)
➤ Authority is the power to hold people accountable for their actions
➤ Positions in the firm should be held based on performance, not on social contacts.
➤ The duties of a position are clearly identified so that people know what is expected of them.
➤ Lines of authority should be clearly identified such that workers know who reports to who.
➤ Rules, standard operating procedures, and the norms guide the firm's operations.

PARETO PRINCIPLE (JOSEPH M JURAN, 1940s)
➤ The 80:20 principle.
➤ 20% of causes invariably produce 80% of results.
➤ 80% of operating profits generated by 20% of customers.
➤ 80% of operating profits generated by 20% of employees.
➤ This 80:20 principle applies to many areas of life.

HAWTHORNE STUDIES (1924–32)
➤ Shift of management theory away from pure mechanistic and economic views of worker motivation and recognition that social relationships could be a greater motivator.

➤ Work groups influence individual worker output.
➤ Supervisors' attention has significant influence on productivity.

MANAGEMENT BY OBJECTIVES (PETER DRUCKER, 1954)

➤ Focus on results not on activities.
➤ Progress towards objectives should be monitored regularly.
➤ Objectives should be SMART: specific, measurable, achievable, realistic and time-related.

THEORY X, THEORY Y (DOUGLAS McGREGOR, 1960)

Theory X managers believe:
➤ the average employee dislikes work and will avoid it
➤ most employees must be coerced and closely supervised
➤ most employees have little ambition and are mostly interested in job security
➤ most employees avoid responsibilities.

Theory Y managers believe:
➤ physical and mental effort in work is as neutral as play or rest
➤ most people prefer to exercise self-direction and self-control
➤ people learn, when encouraged, to accept and seek responsibilities
➤ people are interested in displaying imagination, ingenuity and creativity to solve organisational problems.

MASLOW'S HIERARCHY OF NEEDS (ABRAHAM MASLOW, 1943)

Range from lowest physiological needs to highest self-actualisation needs:
➤ physiological needs, e.g. basic pay, canteen
➤ security needs, e.g. job security, pension
➤ social needs, e.g. teamwork
➤ esteem needs, e.g. company car, new job title
➤ self-actualisation, e.g. more responsibility.

TWO-FACTOR THEORY (FREDERICK HERZBERG, 1959)

➤ Hygiene factors, e.g. salary, working conditions, cause dissatisfaction and addressing them does not motivate employees only causes them to be less dissatisfied.
➤ Motivating factors are intrinsic to the job, e.g. achievement, responsibility, recognition and advancement.

TANNENBAUM-SCHMIDT CONTINUUM (ROBERT TANNENBAUM AND RICHARD SCHMIDT, 1957)

➤ Highlights the range of management style.
➤ One end of the continuum is boss-centred leadership, where there is a large amount of authority used by the manager and little freedom for subordinates.
➤ At the other end of the continuum there is subordinate-centred leadership, where there is little use of authority by the manager and a large amount of freedom for the subordinates.

Manager makes decision and announces it.
↓
Manager 'sells' decision.
↓
Manager presents ideas and invites questions.
↓
Manager presents tentative decision subject to change.
↓
Manager presents problem, gets suggestions, makes decisions.
↓
Manager defines limits; asks group to make decision.
↓
Manager permits subordinates to function within limits defined by superior.

FIGURE 21.1 The Tannenbaum-Schmidt continuum.

MANAGERIAL GRID (ROBERT R BLAKE AND JANE MOUTON, 1957)

➤ There are two variables: the degree of the manager's commitment to achieving the task and the degree of the manager's concern for the people working for them.
➤ Each variable is scored out of nine:
  ➤ 1,1 is 'improvised style', where there is a low concern for achieving the task and a low concern for the people
  ➤ 1,9 represents a low concern for achieving the task and a high concern for people and is called 'county club style'
  ➤ 9,1 represents a high concern for achieving the task and a low concern for people and is called the 'produce or perish style'
  ➤ 5,5 represents a medium concern for achieving the task and a medium concern for people and is called the 'middle-of-the-road style'

➤ the best style is the 'team style' (9,9) where there is a high commitment to achieving the task and a high concern for people.

SYSTEMS APPROACH

➤ Emphasises the interrelatedness and interdependence of the parts of the organisation.
➤ If any part of a system is altered, it is likely to have effects for the system as a whole.
➤ For a system to function effectively, resources such as materials, money, people and information must flow freely through the system.
➤ The desired inputs, outputs and objectives must be identified.

ORGANISATIONAL BEHAVIOURAL APPROACH

➤ Concerns people as individuals, their behaviour in groups, their individual motivations, their development with the organisation and their receptivity to new ideas.
➤ Also takes into account the organisational structures within which people work.
➤ Leaders should try to create an environment in which learning and personal development takes place.

CONTINGENCY AND SITUATIONAL APPROACHES

➤ Recognise that one leadership style will not work for every person, every situation, and every time.
➤ Consider other factors like the flexibility and capabilities of the manager.
➤ Appropriate leadership style depends on the variables present:
  ➤ leader–member relations: the degree to which the group trusts and likes the leader
  ➤ task structure: the extent to which the task is ill- or well-defined
  ➤ position power: formal authority (to hire/fire).

MANAGERIAL ROLES

➤ Roles are characteristics and expected social behaviours of an individual in a particular job.
➤ Mintzberg identified several managerial roles in three categories:
  1 Interpersonal roles: figurehead, leader, liaison.
  2 Informational roles: monitor, disseminator, spokesperson.
  3 Decisional roles: entrepreneur, disturbance-handler, resource-allocator, negotiator.

MANAGEMENT SKILLS

Managers require:
➤ technical skills: to understand how a job is done, what is needed and what is feasible
➤ human relations skills: to be able to deal with people, liaise, negotiate and motivate
➤ conceptual skills: to be able to plan, take an overview and see how changes in one area affect another.

CRITICAL PATH METHOD

Used in project management. The steps are:
1 Define the individual activities.
2 List them in the order they must be preformed.
3 Create an activity diagram or flowchart showing each activity in relation to the others.
4 Identify the critical path – none of the activities in this path can be delayed without delaying the entire project.

ENVIRONMENT ANALYSIS

The environmental analysis is an evaluation of the effects of external forces and conditions on an organisation's survival and growth.

External environment: STEP

➤ Social: changes in consumer lifestyles, tastes and habits affect demand for products.
➤ Technological: improvements in technology affect approaches to promotion and marketing.
➤ Economic: interest rates and levels of income will affect demand for goods and services.
➤ Political: government taxation and laws influence demand.

SWOT analysis

Internal and external environmental analysis.
➤ Strengths.
➤ Weaknesses.
➤ Opportunities.
➤ Threats.

THE FOUR Ps OF MARKETING

1 **Product**: what it does and what it looks like.
2 **Price**: what it costs the consumer, whether there are easy payment terms, discounts.

3 **Place**: whether it gets to the consumer directly from the manufacturer or via intermediaries.
4 **Promotion**: how the consumer finds out about the product and what they are told about it.

BOSTON MATRIX

Divides business units according to their market share and the growth of their market. Business units that:

➤ have a high market share in a fast growing market are called 'stars' and should generally have money invested in them
➤ have a low market share in a slow growing market are called 'dogs' and should possibly be sold off
➤ have a high market share in a slow growing market are usually generating a good profit and are called 'cash cows'
➤ have a low market share in a fast growing market are called 'question marks' and may need to have money invested in them to try to increase their market share or, alternatively, they could be sold.

LEAN MANUFACTURING

➤ Main principle: eliminate waste.
➤ Kaizen: incremental improvement – investment in staff views and ideas leading to a series of small changes that in turn lead to gradual improvement in working methods.
➤ Just-in-time: manufacturing where operations pull required parts at the required time.

THE SEVEN Ss (McKINSEY & COMPANY, 1980s)

➤ Seven interdependent variables within an organisation: structure, strategy, systems, staff, style, skills and shared values.
➤ To change an organisation the soft variables of staff, style, skills and shared values are just as important as the hard variables.

PORTER'S THREE GENERIC STRATEGIES (MICHAEL E PORTER)

➤ Cost leadership based on producing goods at the lowest possible price by producing them in large volumes and so benefiting from economies of scale.
➤ Differentiation involves producing a product with unique attributes that customers will pay a premium price for.
➤ Focus strategy concentrates on a narrow market segment to achieve either cost advantage or differentiation.

PORTER'S FIVE FORCE FRAMEWORK
(MICHAEL E PORTER, 1979)

An industry is influenced by five competitive forces:

1 barriers to entry, e.g. high start-up costs of equipment, patents, distribution channels
2 buyers: their number and power
3 suppliers: their number and power
4 threat of substitutes: willingness of customers to switch, how easy it is to switch
5 degree of competition in industry is dependent on factors, e.g. how standardised the goods are, whether the fixed costs are high, size of competitors.

SUMMARY

➤ There are a large number of management theories.
➤ This chapter is just a brief introduction to some of them.
➤ It is worth learning about some of these theories in more detail.

CHAPTER 22

Mentoring

ONE DEFINITION OF MENTORING

The process whereby an experienced, highly regarded, empathetic individual (the mentor) guides another individual (the mentee) in the development and re-examination of their own ideas, learning, and personal and professional development.

MENTORING

➤ Agenda set by the learner.
➤ Safe place for reflection, listening and support.
➤ Explore strengths and blind spots.
➤ Focuses on capability and potential.
➤ Mentor acts a facilitator.
➤ Discussion of options that mentee has identified.
➤ Typically a long-term relationship.

REASONS WHY SOMEONE MAY WANT MENTORING

➤ Wanting skills to manage change.
➤ Difficulties at work.
➤ Trying to make career decisions.
➤ Issues with work–life balance.
➤ Wanting to develop leadership skills.

BENEFITS TO THE MENTOR

➤ Refreshes own view of work and enhances job satisfaction.
➤ Encourages self-reflection.
➤ Develops professional relationships.
➤ Enhances peer recognition.

BENEFITS REPORTED BY MENTEES WHO ARE DOCTORS
➤ Regained confidence and job satisfaction.
➤ Improved working relationships.
➤ Enhanced problem-solving.
➤ Increased sense of collegiality.
➤ Help in making career choices.

SOME POTENTIAL PITFALLS IN MENTORING RELATIONSHIPS
➤ Failure to establish rapport.
➤ Under-management or over-management.
➤ Poor objective setting.
➤ Lack of time.
➤ Breach of confidentiality.

SKILLS OF A GOOD MENTOR
➤ Good listener.
➤ Discreet.
➤ Able to give and receive constructive feedback.
➤ Able to display empathy and understanding.
➤ Capable of viewing the role of a mentor as a development opportunity for themselves.

FIRST MENTORING MEETING
➤ Introductions.
➤ Length and agenda of meeting agreed.
➤ Clarify expectations (mentor and mentee) and agree what can/cannot be done.
➤ Mentee to give an overview of their experience, strengths and weaknesses.
➤ Agree objectives for the process, i.e. where help is needed, what the mentee hopes to achieve and wants to happen.
➤ Agree process for future frequency of meetings (e.g. two-monthly), meeting place, preparation for future meetings and communication in between meetings (email, phone numbers).

ROLE OF MENTOR IN MENTORING MEETINGS
➤ Establish a relaxed, yet businesslike atmosphere.
➤ Agree the purpose of the meeting.
➤ Explore the issues from the mentee's perspective then do one or more of the following:
  ➢ clarify
  ➢ challenge
  ➢ stimulate

➤ draw on past experiences of mentee and/or mentor.
➤ Summarise.

BEST PRACTICE IN MENTORING
➤ Voluntary process.
➤ Confidential.
➤ Trained, assessed, and supported mentors.
➤ Bespoke matching – mentees are interviewed on the phone to explore their needs.
➤ Careful choice of mentor.
➤ Ongoing evaluation of mentee and mentor experience.
➤ No blame policy – mentees can change mentor if it does not work out.

SETTING UP A MENTORING SCHEME
➤ Obtain the support of key stakeholders and identify the resource implications of the scheme.
➤ Establish the role of a central coordinator for the scheme.
➤ Establish a pool of mentors trained in mentoring skills.
➤ Develop a clear pathway for the matching of mentee and mentor.
➤ Ensure the potential mentees are aware of the scheme and the process of getting a mentor.

SUMMARY
➤ Mentoring can help the mentee have increased confidence and develop new skills and knowledge.
➤ A good mentor is a good listener, discreet, and able to display empathy and understanding.

CHAPTER 23

Patient safety

SEVEN STEPS TO PATIENT SAFETY IN GENERAL PRACTICE (2009)

Step 1: Build a safety culture.

Step 2: Lead and support your practice team.

Step 3: Integrate your risk management activity.

Step 4: Promote reporting.

Step 5: Involve and communicate with patients and the public.

Step 6: Learn and share safety lessons.

Step 7: Implement solutions to prevent harm.[1]

Step 1: Build a safety culture

➤ Carry out an audit to assess your team's safety culture.

➤ Highlight successes and achievements in improving safety, and be open and honest when things go wrong.

➤ Apply the same level of rigour to all aspects of safety, including incident reporting and investigation, complaints, health and safety, staff protection, Significant Event Audit and clinical quality assurance.

Step 2: Lead and support your practice team

➤ Talk about the importance of patient safety and demonstrate you are trying to improve it by including an annual patient safety summary in your practice report or your Practice Quality Report.

➤ Include patient safety in in-house staff training, including the use of improvement methods, and ask for it to be part of continuing education outside of the practice.

➤ Promote safety in team meetings by discussing safety issues and making it a standing agenda item.

Step 3: Integrate your risk management activity

➤ Regularly review patient records (e.g. using case note review tools) so that areas of common harm such as delayed or missed diagnoses/ treatment can be identified.

➤ Keep a good SEA (significant event audits) record that can be used for the General Medical Services (GMS) contract, clinical governance, appraisals and revalidation.

➤ Involve wider primary healthcare team members in improving patient safety and use information from as many sources as possible to measure and understand safety issues in the practice.

Step 4: Promote reporting

➤ Share patient safety incidents and SEAs with the National Reporting and Learning Service (NRLS) so that learning can be disseminated nationally.

➤ Record events, risks and changes, and include them in your annual practice report.

➤ Cascade safety incidents and lessons learned to all your staff and other practices through your primary care organisation.

Step 5: Involve and communicate with patients and the public

➤ Seek patient views, especially on what can be done to improve patient safety, and use complaints as a vital part of a modern, responsive practice.

➤ Encourage feedback using patient surveys and websites such as NHS Choices.

➤ Involve your practice population via patient groups, open meetings or by inviting patient representatives to patient safety meetings.

Step 6: Learn and share safety lessons

➤ Hold regular SEA meetings, reflecting on the quality of your care, patient safety and lessons for the future.

➤ Make the discussion of significant events and the national analyses of patterns of risk everybody's business, including the wider primary healthcare team as appropriate, and act on your findings.

➤ Share experiences with other practices by making your patient safety lessons widely available.

Step 7: Implement solutions to prevent harm

➤ Ensure that agreed actions to improve safety are documented, actioned and reviewed, and agree who should take responsibility for this.

➤ Use technology, where appropriate, to reduce risk to patients.

➤ Involve both patients and staff as they can be key to ensuring the proposed changes are the right ones.[1]

SUMMARY

➤ The Seven Steps to Patient Safety in General Practice are: build a safety culture, lead and support your practice team, integrate your risk management activity, promote reporting, involve and communicate with patients and the public, learn and share safety lessons, and implement solutions to prevent harm.

REFERENCE

1 NHS National Patient Safety Agency. *Seven Steps to Patient Safety in General Practice.* London: National Patient Safety Agency; 2009. Available at: www.nrls.npsa.nhs. uk/resources/collections/seven-steps-to-patient-safety/?entryid45=61598 (accessed 12 December 2010).

CHAPTER 24

Public involvement and patient engagement

Public involvement means involvement in the design, planning and delivery of health services.

Patient engagement means engagement in the patient's own health, care and treatment.

There is good evidence that structured education courses for people with long-term conditions lead to better-informed patients and better clinical outcomes.

Most people agree that involving the users of a service in its redesign will probably produce an improved service.

The NHS is a public service spending taxpayers' money, so it is only right that the public and patients are involved in the governance of GP consortia.

PRINCIPLES OF EFFECTIVE PUBLIC INVOLVEMENT

Be clear about what involvement means:
➤ Have a shared understanding of definitions and purpose.
➤ Ensure adequate resources – money, time and people.

Focus on improvement:
➤ Demonstrate change as a result of engagement.
➤ Embed systems linking decision-making to impact.
➤ Ensure senior commitment and leadership.
➤ Support staff and equip them with the necessary skills.

Be clear about why you are involving people:
➤ Clarify objectives and links to organisational priorities.
➤ Explain what can change and what is not negotiable.
➤ Use what is already known about people's perspectives.

Identify and understand your stakeholders:
➤ Define who needs to be involved and likely to be affected.
➤ Ensure activities are relevant to stakeholders' interests.

Involve people:
➤ Ensure that methods suit the purpose of engagement.
➤ Make special efforts to include seldom heard groups.
➤ Be clear how views will feed into decision-making.
➤ Provide feedback about action you intend to take.
➤ Ensure people have support to get involved.[1]

PROPOSED CHANGES OF THE WHITE PAPER[2]

The NHS Commissioning Board will:
➤ champion greater involvement of patients and carers in decision-making and managing their own care
➤ promote personalisation and extending patient choice
➤ promote accountability to local people for decisions made by GP consortia.

HealthWatch England:
➤ is the independent consumer champion within the Care Quality Commission
➤ will have the power to propose Care Quality Commission investigations of poor service
➤ will work with local infrastructure to provide evidence of needs and aspirations of local communities.

Local HealthWatch will:
➤ provide complaints advisory services
➤ support individuals to exercise choice, e.g. choice of GP practice
➤ be members of local Health and Wellbeing Boards.

Public involvement and patient engagement in GP consortia will:
➤ engage in planning services and considering proposed changes and how services are provided
➤ implement 'no decision about me without me', e.g. commissioning to enable choice
➤ prioritise outcomes.

Patient participation groups in GP practices are:
➤ currently in about 40% of GP practices
➤ important for 'no decision about me without me'
➤ involved in service provision not commissioning.

SUMMARY

➤ The principles of effective public involvement are: be clear about what involvement means, focus on improvement, be clear about why you are involving people, identify and understand your stakeholders and involve people.

➤ The White Paper proposes the formation of HealthWatch England and Local HealthWatch to try to improve public involvement and patient engagement.

REFERENCES

1 NHS and Department of Health, Patient and Public Empowerment Division. *The Engagement Cycle: a new way of thinking about patient and public engagement (PPE) in World Class Commissioning.* NHS and *In*Health Associates; 2009. Available at: www.impressresp.com/Portals/0/IMPRESS/Engagement%20cycle.ppt (accessed 12 December 2010).

2 NHS and Department of Health. *Equity and Excellence: liberating the NHS.* White Paper, Cm 7881. Norwich: The Stationery Office; 2010. pp. 3–6.

CHAPTER 25

Procurement

Procurement is the phase of the commissioning cycle after the service specification when the commissioner decides how to procure the service – by competitive process, or through changing an existing service level agreement. Increasingly, primary care trusts [have been] expected to consider a competitive process, if the investment reaches levels that meet the European Union threshold for an open competitive process.[1]

Commissioners will be expected to demonstrate consistency with the overarching principles of public procurement in relation to all procurement activities. These principles are:
➤ Transparency
➤ Proportionality
➤ Non-discrimination
➤ Equality of Treatment.[2]

ANY WILLING PROVIDER

An Any Willing Provider (AWP) contract means that providers are only paid for the work undertaken. There is no guarantee of any levels of activity and patients should be offered a choice of all providers in the locality . . . The Any Willing Provider model works best under particular conditions which are:
➤ routine elective services
➤ demand is manageable
➤ where there are negligible economies of scale
➤ services where there are low barriers to entry
➤ costs are uniform.[3]

The AWP process is in two stages:
1 The Business Assessment, which tests the providers fitness for purpose as a provider organisation and if passed allows automatic entry (within a given timescale) to future AWP tenders.

2   The Service Specification Assessment, which tests the providers' ability to deliver against the specific tender.[3]

COMPETITIVE TENDERS

'Competitive tender' refers to a procurement process which promotes the use of competition between bidders, in order that the commissioner can seek the best bid and ideally, select the provider who best meets their commissioning need. There are three versions of competitive tender commonly used . . . The three versions are:

➤ Open
➤ Restricted
➤ Competitive Dialogue.[2]

Open Procurement

Under the open procedure, all interested candidates who respond to an NHS Supply2Health® advertisement must be invited to tender. This is similar to AWP but does allow a commissioner to negotiate with bidders and drive down price/increase quality in order to choose the best bid, according to evaluation criteria.

Under this procurement route, the advertisement and service specification must be very clearly defined so that bidders know exactly what is being procured, as well as to enable them to fully assess whether they are interested in expressing an interest in providing the service in question.[2]

Restricted Procurement

Under the restricted procedure, interested candidates are invited to respond to the NHS Supply2Health® advertisement by submitting an expression of interest. A shortlist of candidates is then drawn up and invited to tender. There is no scope to negotiate with tenderers following receipt of bids. This procedure is quite common, because it reduces cost and improves manageability of bids. As there is no ability to negotiate under this route, commissioners must have a clear pricing structure in mind, in advance of advertisement. This is therefore well suited to existing services that require re-provision.[2]

Competitive dialogue

Competitive dialogue is a flexible procedure for use in more complex service procurements where there is a need for the commissioner to discuss all or particular aspects of the proposed contract with candidates. This helps to refine the requirement through supplier input and gives the opportunity for meaningful negotiations.[2]

SUMMARY

➤ Procurement is the phase of the commissioning cycle after the service specification when the commissioner decides how to procure the service

– by competitive process, or through changing an existing service level agreement.

REFERENCES

1 Improving and Integrating Respiratory Services in the NHS (IMPRESS). *Jargon Buster A–Z: procurement*. IMPRESS; 2010. Available at: http://impressresp.com/JargonBuster/ JargonBusterAZ/tabid/63/Filter/P/Default.aspx (accessed 12 December 2010).
2 NHS and Department of Health, System Management and New Enterprise Division. *Procurement Guide for Commissioners of NHS-funded Services*. NHS and Department of Health; 2010. Available at: www.dh.gov.uk/prod_consum_dh/groups/dh_ digitalassets/@dh/@en/@ps/documents/digitalasset/dh_118219.pdf (accessed 12 December 2010).
3 NHS Suffolk. *Commissioning Procurement Policy Appendix 4: Any Willing Provider*. NHS Suffolk; 2009. Available at: www.suffolk.nhs.uk/LinkClick.aspx?fileticket= 55wVIPD%2Femg%3D&tabid=1474&mid=2951&forcedownload=true (accessed 12 December 2010).

CHAPTER 26

Productivity

Productivity is a measure of the output from a production process, per unit of input.

Labour productivity is typically measured as a ratio of output per labour-hour.

RAISING PRODUCTIVITY

➤ Training can improve the knowledge and skills of staff and their ability to produce more.
➤ Ensuring newly recruited staff have a higher knowledge and staff than many of the present staff can result in improved productivity.
➤ Investment in equipment and new technology often raises the productivity of workers.
➤ Employees who are more motivated work harder and produce better quality work.

THE RECOMMENDATIONS OF *IMPROVING NHS PRODUCTIVITY: MORE WITH THE SAME NOT MORE OF THE SAME* (2010)

➤ At all levels in the system the NHS must see addressing the productivity gap as the single greatest challenge in the short to medium term. This will require sustained focus and action.
➤ There has to be a shift from analysing the existing evidence on productivity opportunities to taking action to implement change.

For clinical microsystems

➤ Those in front-line teams, who have the greatest potential to unlock productivity, must reduce variations in quality and productivity at individual and team level.
➤ Emphasis must be given to current initiatives to devolve budgets and manage performance at team level through service line management and GP commissioning.

➤ Key ingredients for a clinical team's success will include:
  ➤ strong clinical leadership and management support
  ➤ timely and accurate information about performance and use of resources including benchmarks.

For provider organisations

➤ Providers must demonstrate strong organisational leadership alongside active personal and organisational support for leaders of clinical teams and directorates to reduce variation in operational service delivery and reduce waste. This will need to include providing robust management and benchmarking information.

➤ Organisations will need to engage and motivate staff at all levels and provide reward and incentive structures for staff that align individual and organisational priorities. Addressing high levels of sickness absence and excessive use of bank and agency staff needs to be part of this strategy.

For commissioners

➤ Leaders within commissioning organisations will need to work hard to sustain focus on quality and productivity and not be unduly distracted by organisational change.

➤ Commissioners need to make full use of the available intelligence and evidence to ensure that they target resources to maximum effect and avoid service duplication. Services need to proactively help people manage their own long-term conditions and avoid unnecessary hospital admissions and interventions.

➤ Integration across health and social care boundaries will be necessary to improve quality and productivity and to deal with the potential impact on healthcare of significant reductions in social services expenditure.

For government and national bodies

➤ Government, the independent commissioning board, and regulators should provide clarity on 'the rules of the game' and ensure that the levers such as employment contracts, tariff, and quality standards are aligned with the productivity agenda.

➤ A careful balance will need to be struck between stimulating competition in some areas of care while incentivising integration and collaboration in others.[1]

SUMMARY

➤ Productivity in the NHS needs to improve significantly over the next few years in order to deal with the difficult financial circumstances.

REFERENCE

1 Appleby J, Harn C, Imison C *et al. Improving NHS Productivity: more with the same not more of the same.* London: The King's Fund; 2010. Available at: www.kingsfund.org. uk/document.rm?id=8723 (accessed 12 December 2010). Reproduced with permission of the King's Fund.

CHAPTER 27

Project management

Project planning brings about the achievement of specific objectives within an appropriate time.

It involves the comprehensive forward planning of all activities.

Effective planning is best achieved when a team adopts a structured approach.

The P-D-C-A (plan-do-check-act) cycle often leads to continuous quality improvement.

PROJECT MANAGEMENT GUIDE

A six-stage service improvement guide for the NHS:
1 Start out: establish a rationale for any improvement work and obtain support for this work from an appropriate sponsor.
2 Define and scope: ensure the project starts in the right areas and develop a project structure to provide a solid foundation.
3 Measure and understand: measure the current situation and understand the level of change required in these measures to achieve the defined aims and objectives.
4 Design and plan: design and plan the activities required to achieve the objectives that have been established.
5 Pilot and implement: test out proposed changes via pilots before the changes are fully implemented.
6 Sustain and share: ensure that changes that have been implemented are sustained and are shared to aid learning.[1]

PROJECT MANAGEMENT PROCESS

1 Agree precise specification for the project.
2 Plan the project: resources, time, team and activities using project management tools.
3 Communicate project plan to the appropriate people.
4 Agree and delegate project actions.
5 Manage and motivate the project team.

6 Complete project and review and report on project performance and praise the project team.

Critical elements for success for a project include:
➤ stakeholder engagement and involvement
➤ sustainability
➤ measurement
➤ risk and issues management
➤ project documentation.[1]

PRINCE2

Prince2 is one standard for managing large projects that has been widely adopted for project management for all types of projects within the private and public sectors.

Within a PRINCE2 project environment, each project undertaken must:
➤ address all the processes concerned with establishing an effective project management environment
➤ have a stated business case indicating the benefits and risks of the venture
➤ demonstrate a properly defined and unique set of Products or Deliverables
➤ have a corresponding set of activities to construct the Products or Deliverables
➤ identify appropriate resources to undertake the activities
➤ have a finite life-span; suitable arrangements for control
➤ identify an organisation structure with defined responsibilities
➤ include a set of Processes with associated techniques which will help plan and control the project and bring it to a successful conclusion.

SUMMARY

➤ Project planning promotes the delivery of specific objectives within realistic timescales through the comprehensive forward planning of all activities.
➤ One framework for project managing service improvement in the NHS is in six stages: start out, define and scope, measure and understand, design and plan, pilot and implement and, finally, sustain and share.

REFERENCE

1 NHS Institute for Innovation and Improvement. *Quality and Service Improvement Tools: project management guide*. NHS Institute for Innovation and Improvement; 2006–10. Available at: www.institute.nhs.uk/quality_and_service_improvement_tools/quality_and_service_improvement_tools/project_management_guide.html (accessed 12 December 2010).

CHAPTER 28

Quality improvement

In 2008, Lord Darzi published *High Quality Care for All*,[1] the final report of the NHS Next Stage Review. The main emphasis of this report was improving quality, which it defined in three dimensions: ensuring that care is safe, effective and provides patients with the most positive experience possible.

The principles of how this will be achieved are:
➤ **Co-production**: implementation should be discussed and decided in partnership with the NHS, local authorities and key stakeholders.
➤ **Subsidiarity**: where necessary, the centre will play an enabling role, but wherever possible, the details of implementation will be determined locally.
➤ **Clinical ownership and leadership**: all staff must continue to be active participants and leaders as the work progresses.
➤ **System alignment**: in doing this work people should ensure that the whole system is aligned around the same vision, allowing them to use their combined leverage at every level to drive up quality.

The National Quality Board is leading on the quality agenda, which is described by a framework pyramid model: at the base are local clinical initiatives to improve services; then provider services will publish quality accounts: then there is the regional activity, to enable benchmarking, using services from the Quality Observatory; and finally, at the top of the pyramid are national priorities and reporting, overseen by the National Quality Board.[2]

INDICATORS FOR QUALITY IMPROVEMENT
➤ A resource of robust indicators to help local clinical teams select indicators for local quality improvement.
➤ A source of indicators for benchmarking.
➤ Assured by clinicians for use by clinicians.
➤ Published with full metadata for transparency.

The indicators are not a new set of targets or mandated indicators for performance management. However, it is possible that some of these may be specified as core indicators to be used in Quality Accounts. The initial indicators are mostly existing indicators that are supported by clinicians and NHS professionals as effective quality indicators.

Clinical governance is the name for the processes NHS organisations use to monitor and improve the quality of the clinical services delivered in their area.

Components of clinical governance:

➤ ensuring effective clinical leadership
➤ maintaining the capacity and capability to deliver services
➤ proactively identifying clinical risks to patients and staff
➤ collecting and using intelligent information on clinical care
➤ involving professional groups in multi-professional clinical audit
➤ involving patients and public in the design of the delivery of services
➤ ensuring the quality of the patient experience
➤ improving services based on lessons from complaints
➤ improving services based on lessons from patient safety incidents/near misses.

SUMMARY

➤ High-quality care can be defined as safe, effective care which provides patients with the most positive experience possible.
➤ The principles of quality are: co-production, subsidiarity, clinical ownership and leadership, and system alignment.

REFERENCES

1 Darzi, Lord. *High Quality Care for All: NHS Next Stage Review final report.* Cm 7432. Norwich: The Stationary Office; 2008. Available at: www.dh.gov.uk/prod_consum_dh/groups/dh_digitalassets/@dh/@en/documents/digitalasset/dh_085828.pdf (accessed 12 December 2010).
2 Improving and Integrating Respiratory Services in the NHS (IMPRESS). *Jargon Buster A–Z: quality.* IMPRESS; 2010. Available at: www.impressresp.com/JargonBuster/JargonBusterAZ/tabid/63/Filter/Q/Default.aspx (accessed 12 December 2010).

CHAPTER 29

Recruitment

Recruitment is the process of having the right person, in the right place, at the right time. It is crucial to organisational performance . . . All those involved in recruitment activities should be aware of relevant legislation.[1]

The following content is reproduced from the Chartered Institute of Personnel and Development (CIPD), UK, website.[1]

DEFINING THE ROLE

Job analysis

Before recruiting for a new or existing position, it is important to invest time in gathering information about the nature of the job. This means thinking not only about the content (such as the tasks) making up the job, but also the job's purpose, the outputs required by the job holder and how it fits into the organisation's structure. This analysis should form the basis of a job description and person specification/job profile.

Job description

The job analysis leads to writing a job description. This explains the job to the candidates, and helps the recruitment process by providing a clear guide to all involved about the requirements of the job. It can also be used to communicate expectations about performance to employees and managers to help ensure effective performance in the job.

Person specification/job profile

A person specification or job profile states the necessary and desirable criteria for selection. Increasingly, such specifications are based on a set of competencies identified as necessary for the performance of the job.

MANAGING THE APPLICATION AND SELECTION PROCESS

There are two main formats in which applications are likely to be received: the curriculum vitae (CV) or the application form. It is possible that these could be submitted either on paper or electronically.

Application forms

Application forms allow for information to be presented in a consistent format, and therefore make it easier to collect information from job applicants in a systematic way and assess objectively the candidate's suitability for the job. They should be appropriate to the level of the job.

Application form design and language is also important – a poorly designed application form can mean applications from some good candidates are overlooked, or that candidates are put off applying.

CVs

The advantage of CVs is that they give candidates the opportunity to sell themselves in their own way and do not restrict the fitting of information into boxes which often happens on application forms. However, CVs make it possible for candidates to include lots of additional, irrelevant material which may make them harder to assess consistently.

Dealing with applications

All applications should be treated confidentially and circulated only to those individuals involved in the recruitment process.

All solicited applications (such as responses to advertisements) should also be acknowledged, and where possible, so should all unsolicited applications. Prompt acknowledgement is good practice and presents a positive image of the organisation.

Selecting candidates

Selecting candidates involves two main processes: shortlisting and assessing applicants to decide who should be offered a job.

Selection decisions should be made after using a range of tools appropriate to the time and resources available. Care should be taken to use techniques which are relevant to the job and the business objectives of the organisation. All tools used should be validated and constantly reviewed to ensure their fairness and reliability.

MAKING THE APPOINTMENT
References

A recruitment policy should state clearly how references will be used, when in the recruitment process they will be taken up and what kind of references will be necessary (for example, from former employers). These rules should be applied consistently. Candidates should always be informed of the procedure for taking up references.

References are most frequently sought after the applicant has been given a 'provisional offer'.

Employment offer

Offers of employment should always be made in writing. But it is important to be aware that a verbal offer of employment made in an interview is as legally binding as a letter to the candidate.

Employers must also be aware of the legal requirements of what information should be given in the written statement of particulars of employment.

Joining the organisation

Well-planned induction enables new employees to become fully operational quickly and should be integrated into the recruitment process.

Documentation

The recruitment process should be documented accurately and access limited to recruitment staff.

It is good practice to monitor applications and decisions to ensure that equality of opportunity is being allowed.

Information should be kept for sufficient time to allow for any complaints to be handled.

Unsuccessful candidates should be notified promptly in writing and if possible given feedback. As a minimum, feedback on any psychometric test results should be given.

CIPD VIEWPOINT

Recruiters also need to be fully aware of equal opportunities legislation and understand how discrimination can occur both directly and indirectly in the recruitment process.[1]

SUMMARY

➤ Successful recruitment depends upon finding people with the right skills, expertise and qualifications to deliver organisational objectives and the ability to make a positive contribution to the values and aims of the organisation.

REFERENCE

1 Chartered Institute of Personnel and Development (CIPD). *Recruitment: an overview.* London: CIPD; 2010. Reproduced with permission of the publisher. Available at: www.cipd.co.uk/subjects/recruitmen/general/recruitmt.htm (accessed 12 December 2010).

CHAPTER 30

Teamwork

BELBIN TEAM ROLES (MEREDITH BELBIN, 1981)

Belbin found the difference between the success and failure for a team depended on behaviour, rather than on factors such as intellect.

Belbin described nine roles needed by a team. Each of the behaviours associated with each role is essential in getting the team successfully from start to finish.

For example, a team with no 'Plant' struggled to come up with the initial spark of an idea with which to push forward. However, once too many Plants were in the team, bad ideas concealed good ones and non-starters were given too much airtime.

Implementer

Is well organised and predictable. Can take basic ideas and make them work but can be slow.

Shaper

Has lots of energy and action but can be insensitive.

Completer/Finisher

Reliably sees things through to the end and ensures everything works well but can worry too much and not trust others.

Plant

Is able to solve difficult problems with original and creative ideas but can be a poor communicator and often ignores the details.

Monitor/Evaluator

Is able to see the big picture and thinks carefully and accurately about things but may not be able to inspire others.

Specialist
Has expert knowledge/skills in key areas and will solve many problems but may be disinterested in all other areas.

Coordinator
Respected leader who helps everyone focus on their task but can come across as excessively controlling.

Team worker
Cares for individuals and the team and is a good listener who works to resolve social problems but may find it hard making difficult decisions.

Resource/Investigator
Is able to explore new ideas and possibilities with energy and with others and is a good networker but can lose energy after the initial burst.

A GOOD TEAM PLAYER
➤ Understands their role in the team and how it fits within the whole picture.
➤ Treats others with respect and is supportive.
➤ Is willing to help.
➤ Is flexible and adaptable.
➤ Communicates constructively and listens actively.
➤ Is reliable and takes responsibility and ownership of their role.

STAGES OF GROUP DEVELOPMENT (BRUCE TUCKMAN, 1965)
1 **Forming**: The group comes together and gets to initially know one other.
2 **Storming**: A chaotic vying for leadership and trialling of group processes.
3 **Norming**: Eventually agreement is reached on how the group operates.
4 **Performing**: The group becomes effective in meeting its objectives.
5 **Adjourning**: The process of 'unforming' the group, that is, letting go of the group structure and moving on.

SUMMARY
➤ Belbin described nine roles needed by a team: Implementer, Shaper, Completer/Finisher, Plant, Monitor/Evaluator, Specialist, Coordinator, Team worker and Resource/Investigator.
➤ The five stages of group development are: forming, storming, norming, performing and adjourning.

CHAPTER 31

Wider determinants of health

Whilst health services make an important contribution to keeping people healthy and helping them when they are ill, there are many other factors which have a direct influence on people's health.

The factors found to have the most significant influence on health are known as the wider determinants of health and include education, employment, housing, crime, social exclusion and the environment.

Figure 31.1 is a simplified pictorial representation of the complex mix of influences and factors that contribute to health.

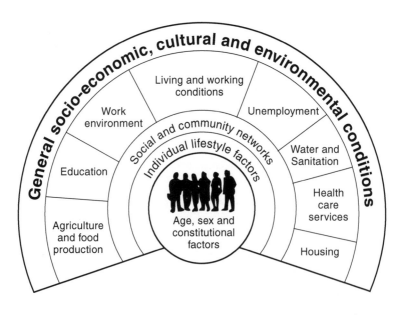

FIGURE 31.1 The wider determinants of health.[1]

Health inequalities are the result of a complex and wide-ranging network of factors. People who experience material disadvantage, poor housing, lower educational attainment, insecure employment or homelessness are among those more likely to suffer poorer health outcomes and an earlier death compared with the rest of the population.

FAIR SOCIETY, HEALTHY LIVES: THE MARMOT REVIEW[1] (2010)
Key messages of this review
1 Reducing health inequalities is a matter of fairness and social justice.
2 There is a social gradient in health – the lower a person's social position, the worse his or her health. Action should focus on reducing the gradient in health.
3 Health inequalities result from social inequalities. Action on health inequalities requires action across all the social determinants of health.
4 Focusing solely on the most disadvantaged will not reduce health inequalities sufficiently. To reduce the steepness of the social gradient in health, actions must be universal, but with a scale and intensity that is proportionate to the level of disadvantage. We call this proportionate universalism.
5 Action taken to reduce health inequalities will benefit society in many ways. It will have economic benefits in reducing losses from illness associated with health inequalities. These currently account for productivity losses, reduced tax revenue, higher welfare payments and increased treatment costs.
6 Economic growth is not the most important measure of our country's success. The fair distribution of health, well-being and sustainability are important social goals.
   Tackling social inequalities in health and tackling climate change must go together.
7 Reducing health inequalities will require action on six policy objectives:
   ➢ Give every child the best start in life.
   ➢ Enable all children, young people and adults to maximise their capabilities and have control over their lives.
   ➢ Create fair employment and good work for all.
   ➢ Ensure healthy standard of living for all.
   ➢ Create and develop healthy and sustainable places and communities.
   ➢ Strengthen the role and impact of ill health prevention.
8 Delivering these policy objectives will require action by central and local government, the NHS, the third and private sectors and community groups.
9 Effective local delivery requires effective participatory decision-making at local level. This can only happen by empowering individuals and local communities.[2]

SUMMARY

➤ The factors found to have the most significant influence on health are known as the wider determinants of health. These include: housing, employment, education, crime, social exclusion and the environment.

REFERENCES

1 Dahlgren G, Whitehead M (1992) *Policies and Strategies to Promote Equity in Health.* Copenhagen: World Health Organisation, Regional Office for Europe.

2 Marmot Review team. *Fair Society, Healthy Lives: the Marmot review.* London: The Marmot Review; 2010. Available at: www.marmotreview.org/AssetLibrary/pdfs/Reports/FairSocietyHealthyLives.pdf (accessed 12 December 2010).

PART 3

Skills needed for effective GP commissioning

CHAPTER 32

Assertiveness

There are three types of behaviour:
➤ aggressive behaviour – I win, you lose
➤ passive behaviour – you win, I lose
➤ assertiveness – I win, you win.

AGGRESSIVE BEHAVIOUR
➤ Aggression is expressing your own rights, feelings, needs and opinions with no respect for the rights and feelings of others.
➤ You express your feelings in a demanding, angry way.
➤ You see your own needs as being more important than others.
➤ The aim of aggression is to win, while ignoring the feelings of others.
➤ Although the short-term effects of aggression may seem rewarding (e.g. release of tension, sense of power) the longer lasting effects are less beneficial (e.g. feeling guilty, resentment from people around you).

PASSIVE BEHAVIOUR
➤ Not expressing your rights, feelings, opinions and needs.
➤ You bottle up your own feelings, give in to others, and see yourself as having little to contribute.
➤ The aim of passive behaviour is to avoid conflict at all times and to please others.
➤ There may be immediate positive effects of being passive (e.g. reduction of anxiety, avoiding guilt, etc.).
➤ However, the long lasting effects may be negative (e.g. continuing loss of self-esteem, stress and anger) and may cause others to become irritated by you and develop a lack of respect for you.

SOURCE OF NON-ASSERTIVE BEHAVIOUR
➤ Often from our experiences of growing up, relationships and life difficulties.

➤ We may have been taught that we should always try to please others and put other people's needs before our own.

➤ We may have learnt that if someone says or does something that we do not like, we should be quiet and try to avoid that person in the future.

➤ If our self-confidence was damaged by being teased at school or criticised at home, for example, then as adults we may be more likely to react passively or aggressively in our relationships and at work, rather than assertively.

➤ Relationship difficulties and experience of loss can cause us to feel that we are unable to take control of our own life.

➤ Low self-esteem and feelings of worthlessness may make us feel guilty about taking care of our own needs.

➤ Although a person may have learned to act in a non-assertive way, they can learn to become more assertive.

ASSERTIVENESS

➤ Being assertive allows you to engage respectfully with other people, whilst also respecting your own needs.

➤ It involves the ability to communicate honestly, directly and openly with other people.

➤ Assertiveness involves being clear about what you feel, what you need and how it can be achieved.

➤ This requires confident, open body language and the ability to communicate calmly without attacking another person.

➤ Saying 'yes' when you want to, and saying 'no' when you mean 'no' (rather than agreeing to do something just to please someone else).

➤ Deciding on and sticking to clear boundaries – being happy to defend your position, even if it provokes conflict.

➤ Being confident about handling conflict if it occurs.

➤ Understanding how to negotiate if two people want different outcomes.

➤ Being able to talk openly about yourself and being able to listen to others.

➤ Being able to give and receive positive and negative feedback.

➤ Having a positive, optimistic outlook.

THE RULES OF ASSERTION – I HAVE THE RIGHT TO:

1 Respect myself: who I am and what I do.

2 Recognise my own needs as an individual: separate from what is expected of me in my roles such as 'wife', 'husband', 'partner', 'parent', 'daughter'.

3 Make clear 'I' statements about how I feel and what I think: for example, 'I feel very uncomfortable with your decision'.

4 Allow myself to make mistakes: recognise that it is normal to make mistakes.

5 Change my mind: if I choose.

6 Ask for 'thinking time': for example, when people ask you to do

something, you have the right to say, 'I would like to think about it and I will let you know my decision'.

7   Allow myself to enjoy my successes: feel pleased about what I have done and share it with others.

8   Ask for what I want: rather than hoping someone will notice what I want.

9   Recognise that I am not responsible for the behaviour of other adults: you are only responsible for your own actions.

10 Respect other people: and their right to be assertive in return.

WHY ASSERTIVENESS IS IMPORTANT

Not being assertive may increase risk of:

➤ Depression: a sense of feeling helpless with no control over your life.

➤ Resentment: anger at others for taking advantage of you.

➤ Frustration: why did I let that happen?

➤ Temper: if you cannot express anger appropriately it can build up to temper outbursts.

➤ Anxiety: you may avoid certain situations which make you feel uncomfortable and you may therefore miss out on activities, job opportunities, etc.

➤ Relationship difficulties: it can be difficult in relationships when individuals can not tell each other what they want and need or how the other person affects them.

➤ Stress-related problems: stress can have a negative impact on the body, and assertiveness can be a good way of managing stress.

BODY LANGUAGE

➤ An important part of assertiveness is open, secure body language.

➤ The way that you hold yourself has an impact on how you are perceived and treated.

➤ Passive body language would be the classic 'victim' stance of hunched shoulders and avoidance of eye contact, while an aggressive stance is one with clenched fists, glaring eyes and intrusive body language.

➤ Assertive people generally stand upright but in a relaxed manner, looking people calmly in the eyes, with open hands.

➤ A good first step to becoming more assertive is to consider your own body language through practising different types of body language (role-playing).

➤ With a friend, or in front of a mirror, try different types of posture and body language as you imagine being the aggressor, the passive 'victim' and finally an assertive person.

➤ See what it feels like to change from being in a passive or aggressive stance to using assertive body language. Just standing in a confident, calm way can feel empowering.

➤ The next time you talk to someone, try to watch yourself:
  ➤ Where are you looking?
  ➤ How would you describe your body position?
  ➤ Is your voice clear and confident?

COMMUNICATION

Clear communication is an important part of assertiveness.
    This is where you show:
➤ Knowledge – you are able to understand and summarise the situation.
➤ Feelings – you can explain your feelings about the situation.
➤ Needs – you are able to explain clearly what you want or need, giving your reasons and any benefits to the other party.

ASSERTIVE COMMUNICATION

It is not just the content of what you say that counts; it is the way you put it across.
    It helps to:
➤ be honest with yourself about your own feelings
➤ keep calm and stick to the point
➤ be clear, specific and direct
➤ if you meet objections, listen to the other person's point of view whilst ensuring that your message is clear
➤ try to offer alternative solutions if you can
➤ ask, if you are unsure about something
➤ if the other person tries to create a diversion, point this out calmly and repeat your message
➤ use appropriate body language
➤ always respect the rights and point of view of the other person
➤ own your messages by using 'I' – for example, it's more constructive to say 'I don't agree with you' than 'you're wrong'
➤ remember, you have the right to make mistakes and so does everyone else.

TECHNIQUES OF ASSERTIVENESS
DESC
➤ Describe the actions or behavior that you see as taking place.
➤ Express why that behaviour is an issue.
➤ Specify the resulting actions or change of behaviour you would like to effect.
➤ Clarify the consequences for failing to change behaviour or meet demands.

Broken record
Simply repeating your requests every time you are met with illegitimate resistance. However, when resistance continues, your requests lose power every

time you have to repeat them. In these cases it is necessary to have some sanctions on hand.

Partly agree
Finding some limited truth to agree with in what an antagonist is saying.

Negative inquiry
This involves requesting further, more specific criticism.

Negative assertion
This involves agreement with criticism without letting up demand.

'I' statements
This can be used to voice one's feelings and wishes from a personal position without expressing a judgement about the other person or blaming one's feelings on them.

PRACTISING
➤ With a friend, practise being assertive in a certain situation, such as refusing to take on extra work, or giving constructive criticism to a colleague.
➤ Explain the scenario to your friend. Using role-play, go through the situation, making your points clearly with your friend responding as the other person.
➤ For example: 'I'd be delighted to help you with that piece of work, but we'll need to agree what other current projects you don't want me to do, because I won't have time to do them all'.
➤ Afterwards, ask your friend to tell you what went well and where you could make improvements.
➤ Try the situation again.
➤ Then swap roles to see the other person's point of view.
➤ Once you have practised being more assertive, think through your new techniques before entering a situation that requires assertiveness.
➤ Imagine your body language, work out how to deliver your message clearly.
➤ Imagine how you will react to any possible responses.

SUMMARY
➤ Being assertive allows you to engage respectfully with other people, whilst also respecting your own needs.
➤ The important parts of assertiveness are: being open, using secure body language and having clear communication.
➤ Techniques are available to improve your assertiveness skills.

CHAPTER 33

Avoiding burnout

One definition of burnout is, 'A state of physical, emotional and mental exhaustion caused by long term involvement in situations which are emotionally draining.'

CHARACTERISTICS OF JOBS WITH INCREASED RISK OF BURNOUT
➤ Lack of control over work.
➤ Lack of control over pace of work.
➤ Frequent interruptions.
➤ Doing a job you have not been adequately trained to do.
➤ Dealing with unpleasant, rude or angry people.

POSSIBLE INDICATORS OF BURNOUT
➤ More irritable and angry.
➤ Decreased concentration and more mistakes.
➤ Feeling shame and guilt.
➤ Feeing emotionally exhausted.
➤ Increased alcohol consumption.
➤ For a clinician, trying to minimise patient contact as much as possible.

MANAGEMENT OF BURNOUT
➤ Diagnose and treat any depression.
➤ Allow time for the person to recognise that there is a problem.
➤ Suggest more hobbies and nice holidays.
➤ Mentoring and support from a colleague.
➤ Suggest they learn new professional skills.
➤ Protected time with family.
➤ Get them to consider early retirement or change of career.

SOME IDEAS TO REDUCE RISK OF DEVELOPING BURNOUT

➤ Talking with family and friends.
➤ Regular exercise.
➤ Doing regular relaxation exercises, e.g. yoga.
➤ Spend time doing enjoyable hobbies.
➤ Get sufficient sleep.
➤ Take regular holidays.
➤ Improve assertiveness skills.
➤ Learn to delegate more.
➤ Improve time management skills.
➤ Have realistic goals.
➤ Have a proper work–life balance.
➤ Avoid excessive alcohol.

Ideas especially for clinicians

➤ Use consultation models, e.g. Neighbour's Housekeeping concept.
➤ Have a short break after a number of consultations.
➤ Develop professional interests different to your main areas of expertise, e.g. dermatology, diabetes, teaching.

SUMMARY

➤ It is important to be aware of the risk of burnout.
➤ Measures can be taken to reduce the risk of burnout and to help those already suffering from it.

CHAPTER 34

Cognitive behavioural therapy skills

➤ Cognitive behavioural therapy (CBT) is proven to be a very effective way to understand and overcome some psychological problems.
➤ In helping us cope with stress, CBT can help us function better in our work.
➤ Quite often the ways we think, feel and behave interact to maintain our emotional problems.
➤ CBT tries to understand this interaction and helps us to make changes in how we think, feel and behave.

CBT can help in:
➤ depression
➤ anxiety and panic
➤ stress
➤ obsessive–compulsive disorder
➤ bulimia
➤ post-traumatic disorder
➤ phobias (e.g. agoraphobia and social phobia)
➤ bipolar disorder and psychosis.

PRINCIPLES OF CBT
➤ The way we think affects the way we act.
➤ Our experiences shape the way we think.
➤ Our thoughts, feelings and behaviour (actions) are interrelated.

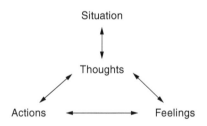

FIGURE 34.1 Thoughts, feelings and behaviours are interrelated.

A vicious cycle
➤ A stressful situation can lead to gloomy thoughts, such as 'I am no good'.
➤ These thoughts can lead to feeling low in mood.
➤ Feeling low in mood can lead to doing less, which in turn leads to having fewer good times.
➤ This leads to further negative thoughts.

Negative thoughts in depression
➤ Tend to be automatic.
➤ Often are biased, unreasonable and unrealistic.
➤ Seem reasonable and correct at the time.
➤ Make depression worse.

Examples of negative thoughts
➤ Overgeneralisation.
➤ Labelling.
➤ Personalising.
➤ Black-and-white thinking.
➤ Jumping to conclusions.
➤ Catastrophising.
➤ Disqualifying the positive.
➤ 'Should' statements.
➤ Mind reading.
➤ Emotional reasoning.
➤ Egocentric thinking.

Overgeneralisation
➤ Words that possibly indicate overgeneralisation are: all, every, never, always, everything, everybody and nobody.
➤ Example: a boy who starts to believe he will never ever have a girlfriend because one girl does not agree to go out with him.
➤ Overgeneralisations are unlikely to be an accurate assessment of reality.

Labelling
➤ Labelling yourself 'stupid' or 'failure' or 'totally hopeless' on the basis of one mistake or one failure.
➤ Can result in seeing yourself only in this way.
➤ Need to understand that one failure or mistake does not make you a failure or stupid.

Personalising
➤ Thinking you are solely responsible for a negative or unpleasant event so you feel unnecessarily guilty and think everything is related to some deficiency or inadequacy in yourself.

➤ Example: 'People are not enjoying themselves at this party because I am not entertaining enough'.

➤ Understand that others may have played a part and you may have only partly contributed to an event.

Black-and-white thinking

➤ Tendency to evaluate yourself, other people and situations in extreme terms.

➤ It is very difficult to meet the stringent demands this thinking can cause.

➤ Examples: 'I succeed at everything' or 'I am a failure'.

➤ This is unrealistic because people or situations are rarely totally one thing or another

Jumping to conclusions

➤ Jumping to a negative conclusion when there is insufficient or no evidence for your conclusion.

➤ This thinking can result in feeling more depressed and less likely to adopt a problem-solving attitude.

➤ Example: thinking you are going to go bankrupt on the basis of little evidence.

➤ Looking for the evidence for and against your conclusion shows when you have pessimistically jumped to a conclusion.

Catastrophising

➤ Blowing a mistake or a fault out of proportion while devaluing the positive aspects of your behaviour or of the situation.

➤ Example: 'This is terrible; I will never be able to show my face again'.

➤ Thinking about how you would view someone in your situation may help you get a more realistic assessment.

Disqualifying the positive

➤ Ignoring positive or neutral aspects of situations and concentrating on the negative aspects.

➤ Also involves changing the positive into the negative.

➤ Example: 'The reason my boss said I have done a good job is because I am incompetent and my boss is trying to get me to improve'.

➤ Thinking about what evidence there is for and against your thoughts may help you reach a more realistic view.

'Should' statements

➤ Having arbitrary and impossible rules for yourself and others.

➤ This can result in guilt and shame with oneself and frustration and anger with others.

➤ Example: 'I should have been able to do that'.

➤ Need to understand that excessively high standards and expectations are not compatible with our all-too-human day-to-day performance.

Mind reading
➤ Where you believe you know that another person is thinking about you in some way and you know what those thoughts are.
➤ Example: 'That person is thinking I cannot do this task'.
➤ Undertand that we cannot read other people's minds.

Emotional reasoning
➤ Believing that if we are feeling something then it must be true, even though we know it is irrational.
➤ Example: 'I feel stupid after making a mistake so I must be stupid'.
➤ Looking at the evidence for and against our feelings will help us get a more realistic view.

Egocentric thinking
➤ Difficulty in believing that other people have a different view to our own.
➤ Example: 'I believe in certain things or hold certain standards so others must as well'.
➤ Understand that other people can have different perceptions and views from us.

COPING WITH NEGATIVE THOUGHTS
1 What is the evidence?
➤ What evidence do I have to support my thoughts?
➤ What evidence do I have against them?

2 What alternative views are there?
➤ How would someone else view this situation?
➤ How would I have viewed it before I got depressed/anxious?
➤ What evidence do I have to back these alternatives?

3 What is the effect of thinking the way I do?
➤ Does it help me, or hinder me from getting what I want?
➤ How?
➤ What would be the effect of looking at things less negatively?

4 Is my thinking realistic?
➤ Am I thinking in all-or-nothing terms?
➤ Am I condemning myself as a total person on the basis of a single event?
➤ Am I concentrating on my weaknesses and forgetting my strengths?
➤ Am I blaming myself for something which is not my fault?

➤ Am I expecting myself to be perfect?
➤ Am I using a double standard – how would I view someone else in this situation?
➤ Am I paying attention only to the bad side of things?
➤ Am I overestimating the chances of disaster?
➤ Am I taking something personally which has little or nothing to do with me?
➤ Am I exaggerating the importance of events?
➤ Am I fretting about the way things ought to be instead of accepting and dealing with them as they come?
➤ Am I assuming I can do nothing to change my situation?
➤ Am I predicting the future instead of experimenting with it?

5 What action can I take?
➤ What can I do to change my situation?
➤ Am I overlooking solutions to problems on the assumption they will not work?
➤ What can I do to test out the alternative views I have arrived at?

SUMMARY
➤ CBT is proven to be a very effective way to understand and overcome some psychological problems.
➤ In helping us cope with stress, it can help us function better in our work.

CHAPTER 35

Conflict resolution

Conflict arises when there are differences among people who disagree about ideas or who find themselves in difficult situations. Conflict over ideas can be desirable and creative when handled constructively.

Situations conflict can cause frustration and resentment if not dealt with. Personal conflict can be damaging and destructive unless it is managed with thought and care. Ultimately conflict can cost a great deal of time and money.

HANDLING CONFLICT SITUATIONS
➤ Do tackle conflict early to keep it from escalating.
➤ Do try to avoid instinctive reactions.
➤ Do think the problem through and plan a way to deal with the conflict.
➤ Do refrain from offering your own opinion before fully understanding the full picture.
➤ Do stay assertive.
➤ Do not avoid the issue and ignore the conflict.
➤ Do not take it personally.
➤ Do not jump in without assessing and understanding the problem.
➤ Do not fight anger with anger.
➤ Do not handle conflict in public.

RESOLVING CONFLICT
➤ Try to get both parties to look at factors which they have in common.
➤ Help the parties to deal effectively with their differences.
➤ Encourage the parties to come up with ways to generating mutual benefit.
➤ Encourage the parties to work out realistic assessments of their point of view.

LEAPS MODEL

Can help you defuse and resolve a potentially difficult situation and also help to bring a sense of professionalism when applied in the workplace:

Listen
Empathise
Ask questions
Paraphrase
Summarise.

FIVE-STEP APPEAL MODEL

Used to de-escalate conflict and is useful when resolving a difficult situation or where a person refuses to comply with a request.

1 Ethical appeal.
   ➤ Make a reasonable request of somebody.
2 Reasoned appeal.
   ➤ The reason/understanding as to why you are making the request.
3 Personal appeal.
   ➤ Appeal to their better nature.
4 Practical appeal.
   ➤ The last chance to get the person to stop what they are doing.
   ➤ Offer alternatives/options/consequences.
5 Action.
   ➤ Make sure you do what you said you are going to do, do not make threats.

SUMMARY

➤ Conflict arises when there are differences among people who disagree about ideas or who find themselves in difficult situations.
➤ Conflict over ideas can be desirable and creative when handled constructively.

CHAPTER 36

Communication skills

Communication is the conveying of ideas and feelings. Effective communication is all about conveying your messages to other people clearly and unambiguously. It is also about receiving information that others are sending to you, with as little distortion as possible.

ACTIVE LISTENING SKILLS

1   Pay attention.
  - Give the speaker your undivided attention and acknowledge the message.
  - Recognize that what is not said also speaks loudly.
  - Look at the speaker directly.
  - Put aside distracting thoughts. Do not mentally prepare a rebuttal.
  - Avoid being distracted by environmental factors.
  - 'Listen' to the speaker's body language.
  - Refrain from side conversations when listening in a group setting.
2   Show that you are listening.
  - Use your own body language and gestures to convey your attention.
  - Nod occasionally.
  - Smile and use other facial expressions.
  - Note your posture and make sure it is open and inviting.
  - Encourage the speaker to continue with small verbal comments like 'yes' and 'uh huh'.
3   Provide feedback.
  - Our personal filters, assumptions, judgements, and beliefs can distort what we hear. As a listener, your role is to understand what is being said. This may require you to reflect what is being said and ask questions.
  - Reflect what has been said by paraphrasing. 'What I'm hearing is . . .' and 'Sounds like you are saying . . .' are great ways to reflect back.
  - Ask questions to clarify certain points. 'What do you mean when you say . . .' 'Is this what you mean?'

➤ Summarize the speaker's comments periodically.
4 Defer judgement.
  ➤ Interrupting is a waste of time. It frustrates the speaker and limits full understanding of the message.
  ➤ Allow the speaker to finish.
  ➤ Do not interrupt with counter-arguments.
5 Respond appropriately.
  ➤ Active listening is a model for respect and understanding. You are gaining information and perspective. You add nothing by attacking the speaker or otherwise putting him or her down.
  ➤ Be candid, open and honest in your response.
  ➤ Assert your opinions respectfully.
  ➤ Treat the other person as he or she would want to be treated.

A MODEL OF THE COMMUNICATION PROCESS

At each stage, there is the potential for misunderstanding and confusion.
1 The sender wants the receiver to understand an idea, which has to be conveyed as a message of some kind.
2 The message is encoded by the sender, who structures it into a logical code – language.
3 When the sender is satisfied with the encoding of the message, it is transmitted verbally or in writing.
4 The message passes through the point of transfer from the sender to the receiver.
5 The receiver decodes the message by making sense of the words.
6 The receiver then understands the idea that the sender wants to convey.
7 Feedback is the process of checking and clarification by asking questions and repeating the message to ensure that the encoding and decoding result in mutual understanding of the message.

MINIMISING COMMUNICATION PROBLEMS

Many communication problems can be minimised by the following actions.
➤ Recognise and respond to the needs of the other people concerned, whether sender or receiver.
➤ Use more appropriate language.
➤ Take more time to communicate the message.
➤ Check for understanding.
➤ Ask for clarification.
➤ Give feedback.
➤ Choose a more appropriate time.
➤ Choose a more appropriate place.

CONVEYING MESSAGES

➤ Use clear and unambiguous language.

➤ Check the understanding of your audience and adapt your message to it.
➤ Have a clear idea of what you are trying to communicate.
➤ Take account of prior knowledge and personal circumstances of your audience.
➤ Use the appropriate level of jargon.
➤ Choose the most appropriate medium to communicate.

SKILLS FOR GOOD INTERPERSONAL COMMUNICATION
➤ Listen with genuine interest.
➤ Be encouraging.
➤ Show understanding and empathy.
➤ Check current understanding.
➤ Reflect/summarise and paraphrase answers.
➤ Use open questions for explorations.
➤ Use closed questions for clarification.
➤ Give information in clear simple terms and use repetition.

FACTS, FEELING, VALUES AND OPINIONS
Albrecht and Boshear in 1974 suggested that in all social interactions, communication occurs through four separate channels: facts, feelings, values and opinions.
1 Facts are real and objective.
2 Feelings are our emotional responses to situations.
3 Values are the norms that exist in society at large.
4 Opinions are our ideas about particular issues, events or situations.

All four channels are used when we communicate. It is important to maintain a clear distinction between them both in your thinking and in your decoding of other people's messages.
    One way to deal with a tense meeting is to:
➤ establish the facts first
➤ invite opinions on the facts
➤ respect feelings, allowing them to be aired but not to dominate discussion
➤ restate common values.

SUMMARY
➤ Effective communication is about conveying your messages to other people clearly and unambiguously.
➤ In all social interactions, communication occurs through four separate channels: facts, feelings, values and opinions.

CHAPTER 37

Consultation skills

Consultation skills can be useful in dealing with interactions even outside the consulting room.

THE CONSULTATION

➤ The consultation is the central task of general practice.
➤ Consultations skills form the basis of good patient care.
➤ Consultations skills can be learnt by systematic training.
➤ Various models have been used to describe what happens in a consultation.

Physical, psychological and social (Royal College of General Practitioners, 1972)

➤ This model encourages the doctor to extend their thinking practice beyond the purely organic approach to patients.
➤ It includes the patient's emotional, family, social and environmental circumstances.

Description of events occurring in a consultation (after Byrne and Long, 1976)

Bryne and Long identified six phases that form a logical structure to the consultation.

1 The doctor establishes a relationship with the patient.
2 The doctor either attempts to discover, or actually discovers, the reason for the patient's attendance.
3 The doctor conducts a verbal or physical examination, or both.
4 The doctor, or the doctor and the patient together, or the patient (in that order of probability) considers the condition.
5 The doctor, and occasionally the patient, details treatment or further investigation.
6 The consultation is terminated – usually by the doctor.

Expansion to include preventative care (Stott and Davies, 1979)

Stott and Davies described four areas that could be systematically explored each time a patient consults:

➤ management of presenting problems
➤ management of continuing problems
➤ modification of help-seeking behaviour
➤ opportunistic health promotion.

Helman's 'Folk Model' (Cecil Helman, 1981)

A patient with a problem comes to a doctor seeking answers to six questions:

1 What has happened?
2 Why has it happened?
3 Why to me?
4 Why now?
5 What would happen if nothing was done about it?
6 What should I do about it or whom should I consult for further help?

Pendleton (1984)

Lists seven tasks that form an effective consultation. The model emphasises the importance of the patient's view and understanding of the problem.

1 To define the reasons for the patient's attendance, including:
  ➣ the nature and history of the problem
  ➣ their cause
  ➣ the patient's ideas, concerns and expectations
  ➣ the effects of the problem.
2 To consider other problems:
  ➣ continuing problems
  ➣ at-risk factors.
3 To choose with the patient an appropriate action for each problem.
4 To achieve a shared understanding of the problems with the patient.
5 To involve the patient in the management plan and encourage them to accept appropriate responsibility.
6 To use time and resources appropriately.
7 To establish or maintain a relationship with the patient which helps to achieve the other tasks.

Neighbour (1987)

Connecting: Have we got a rapport?
Summarising: Can I demonstrate to the patient I have understood why they have come?
Handing over: Has the patient accepted the management plan we agreed?
Safety netting: Have I anticipated all likely outcomes?
Housekeeping: Am I in good enough shape for the next patient?

Six categories of intervention (Heron, 1975)

1 Prescriptive: instructions or advice – directive.
2 Informative: explaining and giving information.
3 Confronting: giving feedback to the patient on their behaviour or attitude, in order to help them see what is happening.
4 Cathartic: helping the patient to release their emotions.
5 Catalytic: encouraging the patient to explore their own feelings and reasons for behaviour.
5 Supportive: encouraging the patient's self-worth, e.g. by giving approval.

Transactional analysis (Berne, 1964)

➤ It explores our behaviour within relationships.
➤ It identifies three 'ego-states' – Parent, Adult and Child – anyone of which an individual could be experiencing at any time.
➤ It looks at the implications and reasons for the different states.
➤ It also explores 'the games people play', which can be used to identify why transactions repeatedly go wrong.
➤ This model is useful for exploring consultations by looking at the relationship between the doctor and the patient.

Balint (1950s)

Explored the importance and identification of psychological problems and identified that many patients' illnesses are distress that do not fit into a disease pigeon hole and suggested the following concepts:
➤ 'The doctor as the drug'. The 'pharmacology' of the doctor as a treatment.
➤ 'The child as the presenting complaint'. The patient may offer another person as the problem when there are underlying psychosocial problems.
➤ 'Elimination by appropriate physical examination'. This may reinforce the patient's belief that his symptoms (neurotic in origin) are in fact due to physical illness. Repeated investigations perpetuate this cycle.
➤ 'Collusion of anonymity'. Referral reinforces mistaken belief in the origin of symptoms. The responsibility of uncovering underlying psycho-social problems becomes increasingly diluted by repeated referral, with nobody taking final responsibility.
➤ 'The Mutual Investment Company'. This is formed and managed by the doctor and the patient. 'Clinical illnesses' are episodes in a long relationship and represent 'offers' of problems (physical and psycho-social) to the doctor.
➤ 'The flash'. The point in the consultation when the real reason of the 'offer' (underlying psycho-social and neurotic illness) is suddenly apparent to both doctor and patient. This forms a fulcrum for change.

Calgary-Cambridge (1996)

➤ Initiating the session – establishing initial rapport, identifying the reason(s) for the patient's attendance.
➤ Gathering information – exploration of problems, understanding the patient's perspective, providing structure to the consultation.
➤ Building the relationship – developing rapport, involving the patient.
➤ Explanation and planning – providing the correct amount and type of information, aiding accurate recall and understanding, achieving a shared understanding: incorporating the patient's perspective, planning: shared decision-making.
➤ Closing the session.

SUMMARY

➤ Consultation skills are also useful for non-patient interactions.
➤ Finding out someone's ideas, concerns and expectations is often helpful.
➤ Transactional analysis can also help us understand some of our interactions and give suggestions as to how they can be improved.

CHAPTER 38

Dealing with difficult colleagues

WHY ARE SOME COLLEAGUES PERCEIVED AS 'DIFFICULT'?

There are many possible reasons for colleagues seeming 'difficult'.

➤ They are stressed themselves:
  ➢ they are having a relationship problem with a member of their own family
  ➢ someone in their family is ill
  ➢ they have money or other problems
  ➢ they are under pressure to meet targets
  ➢ they are tired due to lack of sleep because they have young children at home
  ➢ they are just having a bad day.
➤ They have poor social skills.
➤ They have very high expectations.
➤ They are ill themselves:
  ➢ physical illness causing pain and distress
  ➢ psychological illness, e.g. depression, anxiety, burnout
  ➢ addiction, e.g. alcohol, drugs.
➤ Personality clashes: you find them difficult but most people get on with them fine.
➤ Cultural differences: they were treated the same way in the past and they think it is correct behaviour.
➤ They have learned that they benefit from this behaviour:
  ➢ it enables them to get away with doing less work
  ➢ it gives them a feeling of importance and power.

WHAT ARE SOME OF YOUR OPTIONS?

➤ Ignore the behaviour, be polite and minimise contact.
➤ Confront them in an assertive way.
➤ Speak to colleagues, family and friends to get social support, allies and ideas.

➤ Keep a written record of the behaviour.
➤ Improve your communication and assertiveness skills.
➤ Try to minimise the effect the colleague has on you and do things to reduce your stress level.
➤ Make a verbal or written complaint about their behaviour to your boss.

WHAT YOU DO DEPENDS UPON:

➤ the power difference between you and the 'difficult' colleague
➤ the amount of contact you have with your 'difficult' colleague
➤ the effect the behaviour is having on you
➤ whether your colleagues agree with your opinion
➤ how many allies can you get on your side
➤ whether patient care is affected.

SUMMARY

➤ Consider the possible reasons why a colleague could be 'difficult'.
➤ Speak to people you trust, think through your options and the advantages and disadvantages of each option.
➤ Make a considered plan of action.

CHAPTER 39

Emotional Bank Account

➤ A metaphor devised by Stephen Covey that describes the amount of trust that has been built up in a relationship.[1]
➤ Just as with any bank account, we can make deposits and withdrawals.
➤ However, instead of dealing with units of monetary value, we deal with emotional units.
➤ The emotional units that Covey speaks of are centred on trust.

Positive Emotional Bank Account

➤ Relationships need continuing deposits to sustain a large reserve of trust especially for those people we have regular interactions with.
➤ When we make emotional deposits into someone's bank account, their fondness, trust, and confidence in us grows and our relationship develops and grows.
➤ If we can keep a positive reserve in our relationships, by making regular deposits, there will be greater tolerance for our mistakes and we will enjoy open communication with that person.

Overdrawn Emotional Bank Account

➤ Actions which cause withdrawals include discourtesy, disrespect, overreacting and betraying trust.
➤ When we make withdrawals and our balance becomes low or even overdrawn then bitterness, mistrust and discord develops.
➤ If we are to salvage the relationship, we must make even greater conscious efforts to make regular deposits.

SIX MAJOR DEPOSITS

1 Understanding the individual.
2 Attending to the little things.
3 Keeping commitments.
4 Clarifying expectations.
5 Showing personal integrity.

6   Apologising sincerely when you make a withdrawal.

1 Understanding the individual

➤ Really seeking to understand another person is probably one of the most important deposits you can make, and it is the key to every other deposit.

➤ You simply do not know what constitutes a deposit to another person until you understand them.

➤ What might be a deposit for you might be perceived as a withdrawal by someone else if it does not touch their interests or needs.

2 Attending to the little things

➤ Little courtesies, kind words and warm smiles are at the heart of the little things that brighten up a relationship.

➤ It shows recognition and an awareness of others.

➤ Small discourtesies, little unkindnesses, little forms of disrespect make large withdrawals.

➤ Within our relationships, if you want success, it is the little things that really become the big things.

3 Keeping commitments

➤ Keeping a commitment or a promise is a major deposit.

➤ Breaking a commitment or promise is a major withdrawal.

➤ There is probably not a more massive withdrawal than to make a promise that is important to someone and then not to come through – the next time you make a promise, they will not believe you.

4 Clarifying expectations

➤ A lot of relationship difficulties are caused by conflicting or ambiguous expectations about each other's roles and goals.

➤ It is very frustrating in a relationship not understanding what is expected of you.

➤ Each of us sees life differently and has had different backgrounds and life experiences so may have different expectations.

➤ Many expectations are implicit.

➤ Fulfilling expectations makes deposits in a relationship and violating expectations makes withdrawals.

➤ It is important to make the expectations clear and explicit.

5 Showing personal integrity

➤ Personal integrity generates trust and is the basis of many different kinds of deposit.

➤ Lack of integrity can undermine almost any other effort to create high trust accounts.

➤ Integrity includes but goes beyond honesty.

➤ Integrity involves keeping promises and fulfilling expectations.
➤ Integrity involves treating everyone by the same set of principles.
➤ One way to manifest integrity is to be loyal to those who are not present.

6 Apologising sincerely when you make a withdrawal

➤ When we make withdrawals from the Emotional Bank Account, we need to apologise and we need to do it sincerely.
➤ Knowing when you are wrong and admitting your mistakes prevents the wounds that you have caused in others from festering and allows them to heal.
➤ Sincere apologies make deposits.
➤ Repeating the same mistakes over and over again and then apologising will probably be interpreted as insincerity and will be a withdrawal.

SUMMARY

➤ The Emotional Bank Account is a very useful metaphor for helping to improve relationships.
➤ We can build trust by understanding the individual, attending to the little things, keeping commitments, clarifying expectations, showing personal integrity and by apologising sincerely when we make a withdrawal.

REFERENCE

1 Covey S. *The 7 Habits of Highly Effective People*. London: Simon and Schuster; 1989.

CHAPTER 40

Emotional competence

EMOTIONAL INTELLIGENCE AND EMOTIONAL COMPETENCE

➤ Emotional intelligence determines our potential for learning the practical skills based on our ability to manage ourselves and our relationships with others.

➤ Emotional competence shows how much of that potential we have translated into on-the-job capabilities.

➤ Emotional competence is more important than intelligent quotient (IQ) in determining success at work.

➤ Emotional competence is not fixed like IQ.

➤ We all have strengths and weaknesses over the range of emotional competencies.

➤ We can all improve our emotional competence.

EMOTIONAL COMPETENCIES

Personal competencies – these competences determine how we manage ourselves.

➤ Self-awareness – knowing one's internal states, preferences, resources and intuitions.

➤ Self-regulation – managing one's internal states, impulses and resources.

➤ Motivation – emotional tendencies that guide or facilitate reaching goals.

Social competencies – these competences determine how we handle relationships.

➤ Empathy – awareness of others' feelings, needs and concerns.

➤ Social skills – adeptness at inducing desirable responses in others.

Self-awareness

➤ Emotional awareness – recognising one's emotions and their effects.

➤ Accurate self-assessment – knowing one's strengths and limits.

➤ Self-confidence – a strong sense of one's self-worth and capabilities.

Self-awareness research

➤ Accurate self-assessment was associated with superior performance among several hundred managers from 12 different organisations (Boyatzis, 1982).
➤ A 60-year study of 1000 people with a high IQ followed from childhood through retirement, those most self-confident in their early years were most successful in their careers (Holahan *et al.*, 1995).

Self-regulation

➤ Self-control – keeping disruptive emotions and impulses in check.
➤ Trustworthiness – maintaining standards of honesty and integrity.
➤ Conscientiousness – taking responsibility for personal performance.
➤ Adaptability – flexibility in handling change.
➤ Innovation – being comfortable with novel ideas, approaches and new information.

Self-regulation research

➤ Impulsive boys are three to six times as likely to be violent as adolescents, and impulsive girls are three times more likely to get pregnant in adolescence (Block, 1995).
➤ Children's abilities to handle frustration, control emotions and get along with other people are a better predictor of success than IQ.
➤ Outstanding effectiveness in jobs ranging from semi-skilled labour to sales and management depend on conscientiousness (Barrick *et al.*, 1991).
➤ Primary causes of derailed careers in executives involve deficits in emotional competence. The three primary ones are difficulty in handling change, not being able to work well in a team and poor interpersonal relations (The Centre for Creative Leadership, 1994).

Motivation

➤ Achievement drive – striving to improve or meet a standard of excellence.
➤ Commitment – aligning with the goals of the group or organisation.
➤ Initiative – readiness to act on opportunities.
➤ Optimism – persistence in pursuing goals despite obstacles and setbacks.

Motivation research

➤ Optimism is a skill that can be taught. Optimists are more motivated, more successful, have higher levels of achievement, plus significantly better physical and mental health (Seligman, 1991).
➤ In an analysis of 286 studies from organisations in 21 countries, the achievement motive was the single most frequent distinguishing competence among executives who had superior performance (Spence *et al.*).

Empathy

➤ Understanding others – sensing others' feelings and perspectives, and taking an active interest in their concerns.
➤ Developing others – sensing others' development needs and bolstering their abilities.
➤ Service orientation – anticipating, recognising, and meeting customers' needs.
➤ Leveraging diversity – cultivating opportunities through different kinds of people.
➤ Political awareness – reading a group's emotional currents and power relationships.

Empathy research

➤ Having positive expectations of poorly performing sailors resulted in them improving their overall performance (Crawford, 1980).
➤ An open, trusting relationship is the foundation of success in on-the-job coaching (Peterson *et al.*, 1996).
➤ People who accurately perceive others' emotions are better able to handle changes and build stronger social networks.

Social skills

➤ Influence – wielding effective tactics for persuasion.
➤ Communication – listening openly and sending convincing messages.
➤ Conflict management – negotiating and resolving disagreements.
➤ Leadership – inspiring and guiding individuals and groups.
➤ Change catalyst – initiating or managing change.
➤ Building bonds – nurturing instrumental relationships.
➤ Collaboration and cooperation – working with others towards shared goals.
➤ Team capabilities – creating group synergy in pursuing collective goals.

Social skills research

➤ Between 85% and 95% of the difference between a 'good leader' and an 'excellent leader' is due to emotional competence.[1]
➤ Primary care doctors in the US who had never been sued were shown to be far better communicators than those who had been sued (Levinson, 1997).
➤ Social and emotional abilities were four times more important than IQ in determining professional success and prestige.

IMPROVING EMOTIONAL COMPETENCIES

➤ This requires the retuning of neuronal pathways that run from the limbic centres to the prefrontal lobes.
➤ The person has to weaken an existing habit and replace it with a better one.
➤ There is the need to practise again and again until the new behaviour becomes automatic and spontaneous.
➤ This requires a lot of practice and support.

GUIDELINES FOR EMOTIONAL COMPETENCE TRAINING

➤ Assess the job.
➤ Assess the individual.
➤ Deliver assessments with care.
➤ Gauge readiness.
➤ Motivate.
➤ Make change self-directed.
➤ Focus on clear, manageable goals.
➤ Prevent relapse.
➤ Give performance feedback.
➤ Encourage practice.
➤ Arrange support.
➤ Provide models.
➤ Encourage.
➤ Reinforce change.
➤ Evaluate.

IDEAS FOR HOW TO IMPROVE PARTICULAR EMOTIONAL COMPETENCES

➤ Know your emotions. Work on increasing your self-awareness, the ability to recognise a feeling as it happens. Develop the habit of monitoring your feelings from moment to moment.
➤ Regulate your emotions. Improve your ability to handle feelings and to recover quickly from upsets and distress.
➤ Motivate yourself. Learn to marshal your emotions in order to reach goals. Apply self-control and self-discipline. Practise delaying gratification and stifling impulsiveness.
➤ Cultivate empathy. Put yourself in the other person's shoes. Try to recognise, identify, and feel what others are feeling.
➤ Manage relationships. Respond appropriately and in helpful ways to the feelings of others. Strive for social competence. Hone your leadership skills.

SUMMARY

➤ Emotional competence is more important than IQ in determining success at work.
➤ Emotional competence is not fixed like IQ.
➤ We all have strengths and weaknesses over the range of emotional competencies and we can all improve our emotional competence.

REFERENCE

1 Goleman D. *Working with Emotional Intelligence*. London: Bantam Books; 1998.

CHAPTER 41

Innovation

Innovation: Doing things differently, and doing different things, to create a step change in performance.

Incremental change: Making something a bit better and/or a change that maintains most of the underpinning thinking that is 'the way it has always been'.

Step change: Achieving large gains in performance and/or fundamentally rethinking some of the things that have been taken for granted as 'the way it has always been'.

➤ Both incremental change and step change are useful and desirable.

Innovation means introducing something new into a business. This could be:
➤ improving or replacing business processes to increase efficiency and productivity, or to enable the business to extend the range or quality of existing products and/or services
➤ developing entirely new and improved products and services often to meet rapidly changing customer or consumer demands or needs
➤ adding value to existing products, services or markets to differentiate the business from its competitors and increase the perceived value to the customers and markets.

Innovation is a **creative process**. The ideas may come from:
➤ inside the business – e.g. from employees, managers or in-house research and development work
➤ outside the business – e.g. suppliers, customers, media reports, market research published by another organisation, or universities and other sources of new technologies.

Success comes from filtering those ideas, identifying those that the business will focus on and applying resources to exploit them.

Introducing innovation can help to:
➤ improve productivity
➤ reduce costs

➤ be more competitive
➤ build the value of your brand
➤ establish new partnerships and relationships.[1]

When taking a particular innovative step, consider:
➤ what impact it will have on your business processes and practices
➤ what extra training your staff may require
➤ what extra resources you may need
➤ how you'll finance the work
➤ whether you will be creating any intellectual property that will need protecting.

STEPS TO PROMOTE INNOVATION

➤ Make sure you have processes and events to capture ideas. For example, you could set up suggestion boxes around the workplace or hold regular workshops or occasional company away days to brainstorm ideas.
➤ Create a supportive atmosphere in which people feel free to express their ideas without the risk of criticism or ridicule.
➤ Encourage risk taking and experimentation – do not penalise people who try new ideas that fail.
➤ Promote openness between individuals and teams. Good ideas and knowledge in one part of your business should be shared with others. Team working, newsletters and intranets can all help your people share information and encourage innovation.
➤ Stress that people at all levels of the business share responsibility for innovation, so everybody feels involved in taking the business forward. The fewer the layers of management or decision-making in your organisation, the more people feel their ideas matter.
➤ Reward innovation and celebrate success. Appropriate incentives can play a significant role in encouraging staff to think creatively.
➤ Look for imagination and creativity when recruiting new employees.[1]

SUMMARY

➤ Innovation is doing things differently and doing different things to create a step change in performance.
➤ Steps can be taken to promote innovation.

REFERENCE

1 Business Link. *Use Innovation to Grow Your Business*. Business Link; 2009. Available at: www.businesslink.gov.uk/bdotg/action/detail?r.s=sc&r.l1=1073858796&r.lc=en&r. l3=1074027604&r.l2=1074298365&r.i=1073792537&type=RESOURCES&itemId= 1073792538&r.t=RESOURCES (accessed 13 December 2010). ©2009 Crown copyright. Reproduced with the permission of the Controller of HMSO and the Queen's Printer for Scotland.

CHAPTER 42

Media skills

BUILDING RELATIONSHIPS WITH THE MEDIA

Building good relationships with the media can be invaluable for your organisation. It can help you boost your reputation and get the message across to your key audiences.

Also, in times of crisis or when there is adverse media coverage, having an established relationship with journalists can increase your chances of having your side of the story reported fairly.

So whether the journalist is looking for background information, sound bites for breaking news coverage or a controversial view on a topical issue, it is in your best interests to be prepared.

By building your reputation as a reliable media-friendly source, journalists are more likely to listen to you when you want to put forward your organisation's viewpoint.

Remember, the way and the speed in which you respond to media enquiries will influence the media's perception of you and your organisation.

BASIC RULES FOR DEALING WITH MEDIA QUERIES

➤ Ask for the journalist's name, contact details and media outlet – if you do not know the publication, radio or TV programme or website, make sure you find out more about its audience before answering the questions. It is OK to ask the journalist to send you a link to the website so that you can do some research.
➤ Ask the journalist from which angle they are approaching the story and what they expect to get out of the interview.
➤ Ask to be sent the questions in advance so that you can be prepared.
➤ Make sure you know the journalist's deadline – if you cannot meet it, let them know as soon as possible.
➤ Prepare and check facts and figures and background information for big stories or recurring enquiries.
➤ If you are talking with a journalist about something controversial,

make sure you have a consistent message that is in line with your organisation's views.
➤ Finally, before talking to a journalist, write down two or three key messages you would like to get across in the interview. Try to start and end the interview with these key messages.
➤ Always be helpful, polite and positive.
➤ Remember, you are the expert!

Do not:
➤ use jargon
➤ say 'no comment'. This can sound defensive and the journalist may think you have something to hide even if you do not
➤ talk 'off the record' if you do not want something to be reported. If you speak to a journalist 'off the record', the information can still be used, even if your name is not mentioned
➤ mention facts or information you are unsure about or which you will not be able to source accurately
➤ answer a question if you do not know the answer or if it is out of your comfort zone. You may address the question, but clearly define the scope of your expertise in that particular subject. If possible, i.e. if the interview is for a newspaper or magazine, you can tell the journalist you will get back to them if appropriate
➤ tell a journalist you can help them if you know you cannot.

CRISIS MANAGEMENT
➤ Get your side of the story out as soon as possible. A holding statement may be appropriate while the organisation decides what the next step will be.
➤ Use your media contacts to get your point of view across.
➤ Be honest – address the issue as openly as possible.
➤ Make sure the spokespeople for the organisation are available and fully briefed.
➤ Always include a key message in every answer – regardless of the question.

TOP TIPS FOR RADIO INTERVIEWS
➤ Make a few points clearly.
➤ Use the name of the presenter, other guests and callers.
➤ Do not fidget.
➤ Avoid casual asides even if you think you are 'off air'.
➤ Smile if the subject is appropriate and your listeners will hear it in your voice.

SUMMARY

➤ Building good relationships with the media can be invaluable for your organisation. It can help you boost your reputation and get the message across to your key audiences.

➤ Also, in times of crisis or when there is adverse media coverage, having an established relationship with journalists can increase your chances of having your side of the story reported fairly.

CHAPTER 43

Meeting skills

➤ Meetings can be an important and effective means of both information sharing and decision-making.
➤ However, some meetings achieve little and waste time.

FUNCTIONS OF MEETINGS

Meetings can be to:
➤ bring together a range of knowledge and experience
➤ gather information/give information
➤ take decisions
➤ influence policy
➤ aid problem-solving
➤ develop cooperation and commitment
➤ air grievances
➤ facilitate the evaluation of current activities
➤ explore the effects of current or proposed change
➤ allocate resources.

COMMON THINGS THAT GO WRONG AT MEETINGS

➤ The meeting is unnecessary.
➤ Participants are not given sufficient notice to prepare.
➤ Some participants do not have to be there.
➤ There is no proper agenda.
➤ There is not sufficient time for the meeting.
➤ The meeting is held at inconvenient time.
➤ The venue is unsatisfactory.
➤ The chairperson is not good enough.

SUCCESS OF A MEETING

➤ Meetings succeed in proportion to the chairperson's efficiency and effectiveness.

➤ Meetings succeed to the extent that the participants work as a team and contribute at the level of their greatest capability, knowledge and intelligence.

A GOOD CHAIRPERSON

➤ Clearly states the purpose of the meeting.

➤ Skilfully asks questions beginning with why, what, where, when, who and how.

➤ Distributes the questions so all the participants, particularly give the more reticent participants the opportunity to make a full contribution to the meeting.

➤ Refrains from posing as an authority.

➤ Keeps the discussion to the items on the agenda.

➤ Keeps control of the meeting so that private conversations on the side are curbed.

➤ Makes progress so the group moves quickly down the agenda.

➤ Rephrases contributions in brief and simple language when necessary.

➤ Is good at summarising.

➤ Brings about a cooperative atmosphere amongst the participants of the meeting so the meeting is a team effort.

CHECKLIST FOR MEETINGS

Ensure that:

1. the appropriate people are invited to attend the meeting
2. the participants are given advance notice of the time, place and purpose of the meeting
3. the participants are given the opportunity to contribute to the agenda
4. the agenda is prepared and circulated in advance
5. minutes of the previous meeting and any background documentation are also circulated in advance
6. the environment selected is comfortable and adequate for the purpose of the meeting
7. the meeting has scheduled starting and finishing times
8. the chairperson controls the timing throughout the meeting
9. the meeting starts and finishes on time
10. the agenda forms the basis of discussion, and unhelpful digressions are discouraged
11. no one person is allowed to dominate the discussion
12. all participants have equal opportunity to present their views

13 the participants are encouraged to contribute relevant information and to listen attentively to one another

14 all participants have a voice in decisions made

15 as the meeting progresses, periodic summaries are made of contributions and agreed actions

16 the decision-making process adopted is appropriate to the size and composition of the group

17 the meeting concludes with a summary of achievements

18 any actions agreed on during the meeting are recorded and followed up

19 following the meeting, each participant is provided with minutes or agreed action points.

'PROBLEM' PARTICIPANTS
'Rabbit on and on'
➤ Loves the sound of his or her voice and thinks it is worth hearing.
➤ Response: when the participant pauses for breath, the chairperson should summarise what was said and ask someone else a direct question about another matter.

Openly argumentative
➤ Could be an aggressive personality or a habitual heckler.
➤ Response: the chairperson should honestly try to find merit in one of their points, then move on to something else. If the participant makes an obvious misstatement, the chairperson should turn to rest of the group to let them correct or reject it.

Inarticulate
➤ Lacks the ability to put thoughts into words that can be easily understood by others. Gets the idea but has difficulty conveying it.
➤ Response: the chairperson should say, 'Let me summarise that', then restate their point in clearer language without altering the content.

Having a side conversation
➤ The side conversation may or may not be related to the subject but is distracting to the other participants of the meeting.
➤ Response: the chairperson should call one of the people by name, restate the last opinion expressed by the group and ask their opinion of it.

SUMMARY
➤ Meetings are important but can waste a lot of time.
➤ Measures can be taken to make a meeting more effective.
➤ A chairperson can learn to become more efficient in their role.
➤ There are ways to deal with 'problem' participants.

CHAPTER 44

Negotiating skills

The four steps of a principled negotiation:
1 separate the people from the problem
2 focus on interests, not positions
3 invent options for mutual gain
4 insist on using objective criteria.[1]

In principled negotiations, negotiators are encouraged to take the view that all the participants are problem solvers rather than adversaries. Ideally both parties will come out of a negotiation feeling they have a fair agreement from which both sides can benefit.

STEP 1: SEPARATE THE PEOPLE FROM THE PROBLEM

All negotiations involve people and people are not perfect. We have emotions, our own interests and goals and we tend to see the world from our point of view. We also are not always the best communicators; many of us are not good listeners.

We tend to view people we do not know with more suspicion: Take time to get to know the other party before the negotiation begins.

STEP 2: FOCUS ON INTERESTS, NOT POSITIONS

More often than not, by focusing on interests, a creative solution can be found. It is important to communicate your interests to the other party.

Do not assume they have the same interests as you or that they know what your interests are. Do not assume you know what interests the other party has.

STEP 3: INVENT OPTIONS FOR MUTUAL GAIN

A common problem with many negotiations is there are too few options to choose from. Little or no time is spent creating options.
1 Separate inventing from deciding. Like in any brainstorming session, do not judge the ideas people bring forward, just get them on the board.

2   Broaden the options on the table rather than look for a single answer.
3   Search for mutual gain.
4   Put yourself in the other person's shoes. What things might prevent an agreement and what can be done to change those things?

STEP 4: INSIST ON USING OBJECTIVE CRITERIA

Principled negotiations are not battles of will. There is no winner and you do not need to push your position until the other person backs down.

Use of objective criteria helps remove the emotion from the discussion and allows both parties to use reason and logic. You may have to develop objective criteria and there are a number of ways that can be done, from 'traditional practices', to 'market value' to 'what a court would decide'.

Once objective criteria have been developed, they need to be discussed with the other side.

1   Frame each issue as a joint search for objective criteria.
2   Use reason and be open to reason as to which standards are most appropriate and how they should be applied.
3   Never yield to pressure only to principle.

COMMON CHALLENGES
The other party is more powerful than you

To protect yourself, develop and know your BATNA: Best Alternative to a Negotiated Agreement. The reason you negotiate is to produce something better than the results you can obtain without negotiating.

The result you can obtain without negotiating is your BATNA.

The better your BATNA, the greater your power so it is essential to know your BATNA and take time to make sure it's as strong as it could be.

1   Invent a list of actions you might take if no agreement is reached.
2   Improve some of the more promising ideas and convert them into practical alternatives.
3   Select, tentatively, the one alternative that seems best.

The other party just will not play

In a principled negotiation, you do not want to play games with the other party and you do not want them playing games with you.

There are three approaches to this situation:

1   Concentrate on the merits: talk about interests, options and criteria.
2   Focus on what the other party may do: try and identify the other party's interests and the principles underlying their position.
3   Consider bringing in a third party to assist if steps 1 and 2 are not successful.

The other party uses dirty tricks

The process for dealing with this type of tactic is to follow the process for principled negotiations outlined already. Then, if else fails, turn to your BATNA and walk out.

SUMMARY

➤ The four steps of a principled negotiation are: separate the people from the problem; focus on interests, not positions; invent options for mutual gain; and insist on using objective criteria.

REFERENCE

1 Fisher R, Ury W. *Getting to YES: negotiating agreement without giving in*. London: Penguin; 1981.

CHAPTER 45

People skills

FUNDAMENTAL TECHNIQUES IN HANDLING PEOPLE

➤ Do not criticise, condemn or complain.

➤ Give honest and sincere appreciation.

➤ Arouse in the other person an eager want.

SIX WAYS TO MAKE PEOPLE LIKE YOU

1 Become genuinely interested in other people.
2 Smile.
3 Remember that a person's name is to them the sweetest and most important sound in any language.
4 Be a good listener. Encourage others to talk about themselves.
5 Talk in the terms of the other person's interest.
6 Make the other person feel important and do it sincerely.

HOW TO CHANGE PEOPLE WITHOUT GIVING OFFENSE OR AROUSING RESENTMENT

1 Begin with praise and honest appreciation.
2 Call attention to other people's mistakes indirectly.
3 Talk about your own mistakes first.
4 Ask questions instead of directly giving orders.
5 Let the other person save face.
6 Praise every improvement.
7 Give them a fine reputation to live up to.
8 Encourage them by making their faults seem easy to correct.
9 Make the other person happy about doing what you suggest.

TWELVE WAYS TO WIN PEOPLE TO YOUR WAY OF THINKING

1 Avoid arguments.
2 Show respect for the other person's opinions. Never tell someone they are wrong.
3 If you are wrong, admit it quickly and emphatically.
4 Begin in a friendly way.
5 Start with questions the other person will answer yes to.
6 Let the other person do the talking.
7 Let the other person feel the idea is his/hers.
8 Try honestly to see things from the other person's point of view.
9 Sympathise with the other person.
10 Appeal to noble motives.
11 Dramatise your ideas.
12 Throw down a challenge.

SUMMARY

➤ Make the other person feel important and do it sincerely.

REFERENCE

Carnegie D. *How to Win Friends and Influence People*. London: Vermillion; 1994.

CHAPTER 46

Planning skills

If you fail to plan, you are by default planning to fail.

The six Ps of planning are:

Proper Prior Planning Prevents Poor Performance.

SOME PLANNING TIPS

Set time aside for planning

➤ Think about your entire week.
➤ Plan for the next day the previous evening and your subconscious will help organise while you sleep.
➤ Schedule uninterrupted time every day to do your planning.
➤ Use the first 10 minutes of each day to plan or review your plan for the day.
➤ Each day anticipate the sequence of activities that you will do to attain the objectives you are after.
➤ Take the first 10% of any time block and dedicate it to planning that block.

Major projects

➤ Develop specific plans for how to accomplish major projects.
➤ When starting a new project or activity, take a moment to mentally review the steps you will follow.
➤ List key words that relate to a project. Keep records of how long it takes to do an activity. You can use this information for future scheduling.
➤ Organise information for developing specific plans.
➤ Anticipate possible problems you could encounter in your project because of people, material or mechanical failures. Consider preventive actions and contingency plans in important high-risk situations.
➤ Create and use a Gantt chart. This is a type of bar chart that is helpful in laying out the tasks associated with a given project. It helps to ensure that the individual tasks in a project logically progress.
➤ Put schedules in writing and review schedules regularly.

➤ Set your own due dates for projects earlier than the actual deadline.

OTHER PLANNING TIPS

➤ Do not hurry the planning process. Something will get overlooked.
➤ If you must, leave your office and get away to do your planning in a quiet place where you can think.
➤ Sit quietly and mentally rehearse the steps in your plan. Use your imagination to visualize the steps being taken. You will sense where additional steps need to be added and will anticipate potential problems.
➤ Do your planning on paper to capture all of your ideas and to be sure none of them get lost.
➤ When developing a specific plan, list the activity steps individually on small pieces of paper and then sequence the pieces of paper. Then write the whole plan out in sequential order.
➤ Evaluate plans so that improvements and adjustments can be made.
➤ Schedule formal planning meetings with your staff regularly.
➤ Encourage your staff to create their own plan and then to explain it in detail to you.
➤ Avoid getting sidetracked and losing focus.
➤ Pay attention to details.
➤ Accomplish day-to-day tasks using an orderly approach.
➤ Manage time effectively.

SUMMARY

➤ Proper Prior Planning Prevents Poor Performance.
➤ Schedule uninterrupted time every day to do your planning.

CHAPTER 47

Political skills

The Political Skills Framework: a councillor's toolkit[1] for local councillors has some interesting comments, some of which could apply and be helpful to GPs leading GP consortia.

LOCAL LEADERSHIP
Positive
➤ Engages with their community, canvasses opinion and looks for new ways of representing people.
➤ Keeps up-to-date with local concerns by drawing information from diverse sources, including hard to reach groups.
➤ Encourages trust and respect by being approachable and empathising with others.
➤ Creates partnerships with all sections of the community and ensures their participation in decision-making.
➤ Mediates fairly and constructively between people and groups with conflicting needs.
➤ Acts as a champion for others by campaigning with enthusiasm, courage and persistence.

Negative
➤ Doesn't engage with their community, waits to be approached and is difficult to contact.
➤ Keeps a low profile, not easily recognised in their community.
➤ Treats groups or people unequally, fails to build integration or cohesion.
➤ Has a poor understanding of local concerns and how these might be addressed.
➤ Concentrates on council processes rather than people.
➤ Is unrealistic about what they can achieve and fails to deliver on promises.

PARTNERSHIP WORKING
Positive
➤ Builds good relationships with colleagues, officers and community groups.
➤ Focused on achieving goals by maintaining focus and coordinating others.
➤ Knows when to delegate, provide support or empower others to take responsibility.
➤ Makes people from all backgrounds feel valued, trusted and included.
➤ Understands and acts on their role in building and shaping key local partnerships.
➤ Remains calm and focused when criticised or under pressure.
➤ Is prepared to assert authority in resolving conflict or deadlock.

Negative
➤ Habitually prefers to use status to exert control and impose solutions, rather than involve others.
➤ Fails to recognise or make use of others' skills and ideas.
➤ Finds it difficult to collaborate or work across the political divide.
➤ Prefers to act alone rather than work as part of a team.
➤ Often uses divisive tactics to upset relationships within their group, or council policies and decisions.
➤ Defensive when criticised, blames others and doesn't admit to being wrong.

COMMUNICATION SKILLS
Positive
➤ Regularly informs and communicates with their community using newsletters, emails, phone or local media.
➤ Listens to others, checks for understanding and adapts their own style when necessary.
➤ Creates opportunities to communicate with different sectors, including vulnerable and hard to reach groups.
➤ Speaks confidently in public – avoids the use of jargon or 'council speak'.
➤ Provides regular feedback to people, keeping them informed and managing expectations.
➤ Speaks and writes clearly, using appropriate language.

Negative
➤ Slow to respond to others, communicating only when necessary.
➤ Doesn't listen when people are speaking and uses inappropriate or insensitive language.
➤ Communicates in a dogmatic and inflexible way.
➤ Unwilling to deliver unpopular messages, uses information dishonestly to discredit others.

➤ Doesn't take part in meetings and lacks confidence when speaking in public.

➤ Presents confused arguments using poor language and style.

POLITICAL UNDERSTANDING
Positive

➤ Clearly represents the group's views and values through their decisions and actions.

➤ Helps to develop cohesion within the group and good communication between the group and council.

➤ Communicates political values through canvassing and campaigning.

➤ Actively develops their own political intelligence (e.g. understanding local and national political landscapes).

➤ Looks for ways to promote democracy and increase public engagement.

➤ Is able to work across political boundaries without compromising their political values.

Negative

➤ Lacks integrity, has inconsistent political values and tends to say what others want to hear.

➤ Puts personal motives first or changes beliefs to match those in power.

➤ Has poor knowledge of group manifesto, values and objectives.

➤ Fails to support political colleagues in public.

➤ Doesn't translate group values into ways of helping the community.

➤ Shows little understanding of central government policy or its implications for council and community.

SCRUTINY AND CHALLENGE
Positive

➤ Identifies areas suitable for scrutiny and ensures that citizens and communities are involved in the scrutiny process.

➤ Quickly understands and analyses complex information.

➤ Presents concise arguments that are meaningful and easily understood.

➤ Understands the scrutiny process, asks for explanations and checks that recommendations have been implemented.

➤ Objective and rigorous when challenging process, decisions and people.

➤ Understands and acts on judicial role to meet legal responsibilities.

Negative

➤ Doesn't prepare well or check facts and draws biased conclusions.

➤ Too reliant on officers, tends to back down when challenged.

➤ Fails to see scrutiny as part of their role.

➤ Too focused on detail, doesn't distinguish between good, poor and irrelevant information.

➤ Prefers political 'blood sports' to collaboration: uses scrutiny for political gain.

REGULATING AND MONITORING
Positive
➤ Uses evidence to evaluate arguments and make independent, impartial judgements.
➤ Chairs meetings effectively, follows protocol and keeps process on track.
➤ Follows legal process, balances public needs and local policy.
➤ Monitors others' performance and intervenes when necessary.
➤ Seeks feedback for self and looks for opportunities to learn.
➤ Understands and acts on their judicial role in meeting legal responsibilities.

Negative
➤ Doesn't declare personal interests, makes decisions for personal gain.
➤ Fails to check facts or consider all sides and makes subjective or uninformed judgements.
➤ Habitually leaves monitoring and checks on progress to others.
➤ Makes decisions without taking advice, considering regulations or taking account of wider issues.
➤ Doesn't recognise or address limits of own knowledge or expertise.
➤ Misses deadlines, leaves business unfinished and lacks balance between council and other commitments.[1]

SUMMARY
➤ The *Political Skills Framework: a councillor's toolkit* has some interesting comments, some of which could apply and be helpful to GPs leading GP consortia.

REFERENCE
1 Silvester J, for the Improvement and Development Agency. *The Political Skills Framework: a councillor's toolkit.* London: Improvement and Development Agency; 2007. Available at: www.idea.gov.uk/idk/aio/6515699 (accessed 13 December 2010).

CHAPTER 48

Presentational skills

QUESTIONS TO CONSIDER BEFORE PLANNING A PRESENTATION

➤ What is the main purpose of your presentation – to inform, persuade, motivate or change things?

➤ Who is your audience – their number, role, knowledge, interest, preconceptions and expectations?

➤ What to do you want your audience to do as a result of your presentation?

➤ What is the overall message you want to deliver?

➤ What are the main points you need to make to get your message across?

➤ What supporting information are you likely to need and where can you obtain it?

➤ What will be the most informative and interesting title for your presentation?

➤ How long is the presentation going to be?

➤ What is the most appropriate form and level of language for your audience?

➤ What are the likely questions you may be asked at the end of your presentation?

SOME PRESENTATIONAL TIPS

➤ You should rehearse your presentation several times so that you know it well, even without any visual aids. Check beforehand any electrical equipment you are planning to use.

➤ First impressions are very important. The audience will make judgements about you even before you start to speak, based on the way you come across and how you look. They will continue to form opinions about you based on the way you speak.

➤ In order for your audience to take you seriously you need to look confident and look like you know what you are talking about right from the start of the presentation.

➤ Act enthusiastic, make and maintain eye contact, smile, try to look relaxed and to make your introduction without looking at your notes. Project your voice to the furthest member of the audience.

➤ Speak clearly and at conversational speed. Do not mumble, rush your words or use a monotone delivery. This is particularly important if you are reading verbatim from a personal speech. Use the natural inflections of conversation. You may also emphasise key words, which will help to influence the overall meaning of your messages.

➤ Control your audience by maintaining eye contact and by looking for and responding to signs of puzzlement or boredom. Do not bury your head in your notes or use 'fillers' such as 'er', 'um', 'right' or 'you know'. Use pauses instead.

➤ Injecting pauses into your speaking also helps to create an impact as well as helping you to control your speed so that you don't race ahead too quickly and make it hard for the audience to follow.

➤ Avoid distracting your audience with unnecessary pacing around, fiddling or gesturing, and make sure that you keep an eye on the time. Having to rush through the last few points will mean that you will not do justice to your argument.

➤ Lead up to your concluding remarks by signposting the way. Phrases such as 'and my final point is' or 'if I can just sum up my main points' will let your audience know that the end is in sight so they can expect some conclusions and recommendations or a summary.

➤ Finish as enthusiastically as you began. Make sure that your audience has got the message you wanted to deliver and finish on a high point.

SUMMARY

➤ Presentational skills can be improved by rehearsing, making a good first impression, speaking confidently, sounding interesting, looking confident and by engaging with the audience.

CHAPTER 49

Stress management

ACCEPT THE THINGS YOU CANNOT CHANGE

Recognise and accept the things you cannot change and concentrate on the things you do have control over.

AVOID UNHEALTHY HABITS

Do not rely on alcohol, smoking and caffeine as your ways of coping.

BE POSITIVE

Look for the positives in life, and things for which you are grateful.

CONNECT WITH PEOPLE

A good support network of colleagues, friends and family can ease your troubles and help you see things in a different way.

DO VOLUNTEER WORK

People who help others, through activities such as volunteering or community work, become more resilient.

HAVE SOME 'ME TIME'

Set aside enough time in the week to have some quality 'me time' doing things that give you pleasure.

PHYSICAL ACTIVITY

Regular physical activity can reduce some of the emotional intensity you are feeling, clear your thoughts and enable you to deal with your problems more calmly.

WORK SMARTER, NOT HARDER

This means prioritising your work, concentrating on the tasks that will make a real difference to your work.

WRITING DOWN YOUR THOUGHTS AND FEELINGS

This can help to get your thoughts and feelings from the inside to the outside and help you see your problems in a different way.

PROGRESSIVE MUSCLE RELAXATION FOR STRESS RELIEF

This involves a two-step process in which you systematically tense and relax different muscle groups in the body.

With regular practice, progressive muscle relaxation helps you to understand what tension and complete relaxation feels like.

This awareness helps you spot and counteract the first signs of the muscular tension that accompanies stress.

➤ Get comfortable and take a few minutes to relax, breathing in and out in slow, deep breaths.

➤ Once relaxed, shift your attention to your right foot and take a moment to focus on the way it feels.

➤ Slowly tense the muscles in your right foot, squeezing as tightly as you can. Hold for a count of 10.

➤ Relax your right foot. Focus on the tension flowing away and the way your foot feels as it becomes limp and loose.

➤ Stay in this relaxed state for a moment, breathing deeply and slowly.

➤ When you're ready, shift your attention to your left foot. Follow the same sequence of muscle tension and release.

➤ Move slowly up through your body – legs, abdomen, back, neck and face – contracting and relaxing the muscle groups as you go.

SUMMARY

➤ Talking to people we can trust, doing regular exercise and writing down our thoughts and feelings can help us all cope better with stress.

➤ Progressive muscle relaxation is another helpful technique.

CHAPTER 50

Time management

For effective time management, Stephen Covey advises that we should **organise and execute around priorities**.

He divides activities into four quadrants according to their urgency and importance.

Quadrant 1 represents things which are both urgent and important. This can be called 'fire fighting'. These activities need to be dealt with immediately, and they are important.

Quadrant 2 represents things which are important, but not urgent. The activities contribute to achieving our goals and priorities but they do not have to be done right now. Some examples of Quadrant 2 activities are preparation, planning, prevention, relationship building and personal development.

Quadrant 3 activities are distractions. They must be dealt with right now, but are not important. For example, when you answer an unwanted phone call, you have had to interrupt whatever you were doing to answer it.

The final quadrant, Quadrant 4, is activities which are neither urgent nor important.

Quadrant 1 **URGENT AND IMPORTANT**	Quadrant 2 **NOT URGENT BUT IMPORTANT**
Crisis	Planning
Deadlines	Prevention
Child crying	Relationship building
Emergencies	Personal development
	Regular exercise
Quadrant 3 **URGENT BUT NOT IMPORTANT**	Quadrant 4 **NOT URGENT AND NOT IMPORTANT**
Some interruptions	Excessive television
Some mail	Time wasting activities
Some phone calls	Some phone calls

FIGURE 50.1 Covey's four quadrants for effective time management.

Covey emphasises the importance of maximising the amount of time spent in Quadrant 2 activities. Allocate time in your diary to carry out these tasks when you are at your best.

By concentrating on Quadrant 2 activities, the 'fire fighting' Quadrant 1 activities decrease in number. You should also seek to reduce time spent in Quadrant 3 by improving your systems and processes for dealing with distractions. You should seek to eliminate as much as possible of Quadrant 4 activities.

OTHER TIPS FOR TIME MANAGEMENT

➤ Plan and use a weekly to-do list rather than a daily to-do list.
➤ To focus your time on that which is truly important, that is in line with your goals, you will need to write down what you are trying to achieve across the key roles and different parts of your life.
➤ Put personal items and work items on the same calendar.
➤ Clean up clutter.
➤ Look for ways to use commuting time for doing something constructive.
➤ Delegate as often as you can.
➤ Concern yourself with doing the right things (effectiveness) rather than doing things right (efficiency).
➤ Try to minimise unhelpful interruptions.
➤ Meetings can waste a lot of time (see tips in Chapter 43).
➤ Email can waste time (see tips in Chapter 15).
➤ Pick your priorities very carefully.
➤ Avoid procrastination.
➤ Things that are scheduled are more likely to happen.

SUMMARY

➤ Try to increase the time you are doing activities that are important but not urgent.
➤ Organise and execute around priorities.

REFERENCE

Covey S. *The 7 Habits of Highly Effective People*. London: Simon and Schuster; 1989.

PART 4

Attitudes needed for effective GP commissioning

Adherence to the Nolan Principles of public life

People involved in GP commissioning should abide by the Nolan Principles.

Lord Nolan in the *Report of his Committee on Standards in Public Life* set out what he called the Seven Principles of Public Life.

1 SELFLESSNESS

Holders of public office should act solely in terms of the public interest. They should not do so in order to gain financial or other material benefits for themselves, their family, or their friends.

2 INTEGRITY

Holders of public office should not place themselves under any financial or other obligation to outside individuals or organisations that might seek to influence them in the performance of their official duties.

3 OBJECTIVITY

In carrying out public business, including making public appointments, awarding contracts, or recommending individuals for rewards and benefits, holders of public office should make choices on merit.

4 ACCOUNTABILITY

Holders of public office are accountable for their decisions and actions to the public and must submit themselves to whatever scrutiny is appropriate to their office.

5 OPENNESS

Holders of public office should be as open as possible about all the decisions and actions that they take. They should give reasons for their decisions and restrict information only when the wider public interest clearly demands.

6 HONESTY

Holders of public office have a duty to declare any private interests relating to their public duties and to take steps to resolve any conflicts arising in a way that protects the public interest.

7 LEADERSHIP

Holders of public office should promote and support these principles by leadership and example.[1]

REFERENCE

HMSO. *Summary of the Nolan Committee's First Report on Standards in Public Life*. HMSO; 1996. Available at: www.archive.official-documents.co.uk/document/parlment/nolan/nolan.htm (accessed 13 December 2010).

CHAPTER 52

Other attitudes needed for effective GP commissioning

COST-EFFECTIVENESS

With the aging population and the rapid advances in modern medicine, no publicly funded healthcare system can possibly pay for every new medical treatment that becomes available. The enormous costs involved mean that choices have to be made. It makes sense to focus on treatments that improve the quality and/or length of someone's life and, at the same time, that are an effective use of NHS resources.

LONG-TERM THINKING

GP commissioning will have to try to make decisions that are in the best long-term interests of patients and the public. This may mean that some decisions that save money in the short term need to be rethought if the long-term consequences are significant and negative.

OUTCOMES NOT ACTIVITY

The White Paper[1] signals a shift from payment based on activity to a greater concentration on patient outcomes. One effect of this may be that less money is spent on glamorous high-technology medicine and more resources devoted to simple interventions that have been proven to improve the quality of peoples' lives.

PATIENT FOCUS

The Kennedy Report in 2001[2] said patients in their journey through the healthcare system are entitled to be treated with respect and honesty and to be involved, wherever possible, in decisions about their treatment. As patients and the public have greater power in the NHS, this should lead to improved quality of care and less risk of poor care going unchallenged.

PRAGMATISM NOT IDEOLOGY

The NHS has been often treated as a political football in the past. A better approach is to see which policies work to produce results that are in the best long-term interests of patients and the public and which polices do not work. This shift to evidence-based policy-making for the NHS is a better way forward for the future.

TOUGH LOVE

The difficult financial circumstances facing the NHS in the next few years will mean there will have to be some very agonising decisions made about services and jobs.

For the NHS to to be here and functioning well 50 years from now, I believe it is better that the GP consortia provide 'tough love' to the NHS rather than try to ignore the external realities.

COMMITMENT TO CREATING WIN-WIN SITUATIONS

In the difficult financial circumstances ahead, it will be tempting for GP consortia to try to force through contracts that do not take into account the long-term viability of providers. But the contracts that are agreed on will need to take into account the difficult financial circumstances and still maintain the long-term viability of the providers. This balance is difficult but will be vitally important in the years ahead.

REFERENCES

1 NHS and Department of Health. *Equity and Excellence: liberating the NHS*. White Paper, Cm 7881. Norwich: The Stationery Office; 2010.
2 The Bristol Royal Infirmary Inquiry. *Learning from Bristol: the report of the public inquiry into children's heart surgery at the Bristol Royal Infirmary 1984–1995*. Command Paper, Cm 5207. The Bristol Royal Infirmary Inquiry; 2001.

Conclusion

The NHS White Paper of July 2010 has proposed a massive shake up of the NHS in England. The PCTs will be abolished and it is proposed that their commissioning function be mainly taken over by GPs working together in consortia. The difficult financial circumstances that the NHS will face over the next few years will require marked improvements in quality, innovation, productivity and prevention.

The intention of this book is to help clinicians and non-clinicians involved in GP commissioning to gain a better idea of the knowledge, skills and attitudes needed for them to succeed. This book can only be an introduction and to acquire some of these knowledge and skills to the appropriate standard will require time, practise and expert help. The NHS is facing a great challenge in the next few years to justify the trust the British public have in it. I hope that this book will make a contribution to the NHS successfully meeting this challenge.

Index

Page numbers in **bold** refer to illustrations.